Fundamental Aspects of Women's Health

Other titles in the Fundamental Aspects of Nursing series include:

Fundamental Aspects of Legal, Ethical and Professional Issues in Nursing by Maggie Reeves and Jacqui Orford

Fundamental Aspects of Men's Health by Morag A Gray

Fundamental Aspects of Mental Health Nursing by Ben Thomas

Fundamental Aspects of Palliative Care Nursing by Robert Becker and Richard Gamlin

Fundamental Aspects of Child Health Nursing by the Birmingham Children's Hospital NHS Trust

Fundamental Aspects of
Women's Health

Morag A Gray

Quay
Books

Mark Allen
Publishing Ltd

Quay Books Division, Mark Allen Publishing Limited, Jesses Farm, Snow Hill, Dinton, Salisbury, Wiltshire SP3 5HN

British Library Cataloguing-in-Publication Data
A catalogue record is available for this book

© Mark Allen Publishing Limited 2003
ISBN 1 85642 190 2

Printed in the UK by Bath Press, Bath

Contents

Contents

Foreword

There is an old Gaelic saying, Is e an oighreachd an t-slainte' which translated means 'Health is the inheritance'.

(Downie *et al*, 1996)

Health is defined in the World Health Organization's (WHO) constitution of 1948 as:

A State of complete physical, social and mental well-being and not merely the absence of disease or infirmity.

Within the context of health promotion, health has been considered less than an abstract state and more as a means to an end which can be expressed in functional terms as a resource which permits people to lead an individually, socially and economically productive life.

Health is a resource for everyday life, not the object of living. It is a positive concept emphasising social and personal resources as well as physical capabilities

(Ottawa Charter for Health Promotion, WHO, Geneva 1986)

Women's health differs from men's both in terms of its patterns and the illnesses experienced. Although women live longer than men, they report more illness and distress than men. Put simply, this means that women seem to experience a less healthy life than men. However, women have not always lived longer than men. Indeed, it first became apparent in the latter part of the nineteenth century and to this day, the life expectancy of males and females in Southern Asia remains equal and in Bangladesh men live longer than women (World Health Organization [WHO], 1998b). Reasons proposed for the increased longevity of women are the introduction of birth control, providing women with a means of having control over family size, general improvements in living standards and the introduction of maternity services (WHO, 1998b).

In order to understand health, one must consider systems and structures that govern social and economic as well as the physical environment, and take cognisance of how these factors impinge on health both at a social and personal level. This book attempts to provide the reader with a source of fundamental information on women's health. In the past, texts on women's health have been confined to dealing with topics related to reproductive health. This text aims to provide the reader with a broader perspective of health related issues in general and relevant to women in particular.

Morag A Gray
December 2002

References

Downie RS, Tannahill C, Tannahill A (1996) *Health Promotion: Models and Values*. 2nd edn. Oxford University Press, Oxford

World Health Organization (1986) *Ottawa Charter for Health Promotion*. WHO, Geneva

World Health Organization (1998b) *Gender and Health: Technical paper*. World Health Organization, Geneva

Acknowledgements

I am indebted to my husband Chris for his unfailing support and encouragement.

I would also like to acknowledge my colleague, Rhona Elliott, who contributed to this book.

I

The context of women's health

Introduction

Women's health pertains to the physical, psychological and social well-being of women. Sex is innate, but it is argued that gender is socially created and learned by individuals. Being born male or female does not necessarily lead to thinking, acting and feeling in ways that culture prescribes for men and women. As we communicate with others, we learn how society defines the sexes and we craft our personal identities to reflect and resist social expectations. As we enter diverse situations and relationships during our lives, our understandings of gender continuously evolve. Gender is more than a facet of personal identity, it is also a system of social meanings that is constructed and sustained by a variety of cultural structures and practices. These multiple social structures and practices sustain society's gender ideology. Health is a fundamental human right and everyone is entitled to access basic resources for health (World Health Organization [WHO], 1998a).

This chapter serves to place women's health in context. The intention is to cover a broad range of aspects that relate to general aspects of health. The chapter begins with a short description of what health promotion means and what it involves, including a brief reference to health promotion models. The issue of changing lifestyle behaviours is tackled next with links made to the Health Belief Model. The aspect of poverty, unemployment and health inequality is the focus of the remainder of the chapter. A few suggested web resources are supplied for further information.

Health promotion

Health promotion is a term generally used to reflect activities that are employed to prevent disease, improve health and enhance well-being (Naidoo and Wills, 1998). Downie *et al* (1996) add that empowerment is a cardinal principle in any health promotion activity. Liimatainen *et al* (2001) define health promotion as a process of enabling people to increase control over their health and to improve it. A more comprehensive definition is offered by Tones (1991) who divides health promotion into three components: health education, disease prevention and health surveillance. Tones explains that health education is a particularly significant part as the manner in which information is relayed is fundamental to understanding. The 1986 Ottawa Charter for health promotion defined it as the process which enables people to increase control over, and to improve their health (WHO, 1986).

The primary focus of health promotion according to Bennett and Murphy (1997) is to change behaviour to improve health. Paramount to any successful health promotion activity is the concept of empowerment and the absolute requirement for active involvement of the individual concerned. The health professional working in a holistic manner must enter into a partnership with the client, the outcome of which should be a well-informed person who is able to participate in a problem-solving approach to achieve optimum health for them as an individual (Walker, 2000). Tones (2002) reinforces the importance of empowering the person, rather than adopting a victim blaming perspective.

Downie *et al* (1996) assert that in addition to empowering the individual, the power holders in society must also embrace this approach through public health policies which aim to develop life skills and foster self-esteem.

Kendal and Lask (1997) refer to the WHO's (1986) five principles of health promotion, which state that health promotion:

- involves the population as a whole in the context of their everyday life, rather than focusing on people at risk of specific illnesses
- is directed towards action on the determinants[1] or cause of health
- combines diverse but complementary methods or approaches
- aims particularly at effective and concrete public participation
- involves health professionals, particularly in primary health care, who have an important role in nurturing and enabling the process.

---

1   Determinant of health can be defined as the 'range of personal, social, economic and environmental factors which determine the health status of individuals or populations' (WHO, 1998a, p. 6).

Naidoo and Wills (1998) provide four elements of health promotion. Firstly, disease prevention which includes activities such as screening. Secondly, health education and information giving delivered through a variety of media, such as television campaigns, advertisements, leaflets, and websites. Thirdly, public health promotion activities, which aim to improve sexual and environmental health through local initiatives to increase access to services and public health policies. Lastly, community development activities, which focus on individual development of necessary knowledge, skills and social networks to improve their health, for example, through women's help groups. Kawachi and Kennedy (1997) suggest the value of social networks is evidenced in that people with good social support are three times more likely to survive a myocardial infarction than those with poor social support.

There are a variety of health promotion models that attempt to bridge the gap between theory and practice (Naidoo and Wills, 1998). The variety in models reflects the beliefs of the individuals who developed the model. They differ in terms of the theory underpinning health, education, the individual, societal change and the relationship between all these factors (Naidoo and Wills, 1998). Models facilitate our understanding of:

> ... *people's views about the causes of ill health, the extent to which people feel that they can control their life and make changes, how people explain their health and illness, which is crucial in making sense of the strategies they adopt to promote health, prevent ill health and manage illness.*

> (Naidoo and Wills, 2001, p. 86)

The most commonly cited health promotion models are Tannahill (1985) and Eweles and Simnett (1999), which are referred to as descriptive models as they identify the medley of existing practices but make no attempt to judge their value. A model that does make such a judgement is known as an analytical model and the most commonly cited of these is that of Beattie (1991). Naidoo and Wills (2001) describe Tannahill's model as possessing three intersecting circles that represent health education, prevention and health protection. They continue by stating that within these intersecting circles there are seven possible dimensions of health promotion. These are listed as:

- preventative services (eg. screening)
- preventative health education (eg. smoking cessation advice)
- preventative health protection (eg. water fluoridation)
- health education for preventative health protection (eg. seat belt lobbying)
- positive health education (eg. building life skills[2])
- positive health protection (eg. workplace smoking policy)
- health education aimed at positive health protection (eg. campaigning for protective legislation).

Eweles and Simnett's (1999) model, according to Naidoo and Wills (2001), uses five areas to describe a variety of theoretical perspectives relevant to health promotion. They quote Eweles and Simnett as stating:

In our view, there is no one 'right' aim for health promotion, and no one 'right' approach or set of activities. We need to work out for ourselves which aim and activities we use, in accordance with our own professional code of conduct (if there is one), our own carefully considered values and our own assessment of the client's needs.

(p. 283)

Beattie's (1991) model identifies four approaches for health promotion: health persuasion, personal counselling, community development and legislative action for health (Naidoo and Wills, 1998).

Health education can be defined as:

An intentional activity that is designed to achieve health or illness related learning, ie. some relatively permanent change in an individual's capability or disposition. Effective health education may, thus, produce changes in knowledge and understanding or ways of thinking; it may influence or clarify values; it may bring about some shift in belief or attitude; it may facilitate the acquisition of skills; it may even effect changes in behaviour or lifestyle.

(Tones and Tilford, 2001, p. 30, cited by Tones 2002)

The WHO (1998a, p. 4) defines health education as comprising, 'consciously constructed opportunities for learning involving some

---

2   Life skills can be defined as the 'abilities for adaptive and positive behaviour, that enable individuals to deal effectively with the demands and challenges of every day life' (WHO, 1998a, p. 15).

form of communication designed to improve health literacy, including improving knowledge, and developing life skills which are conducive to individual and community health.'

> *Not taking care of your body is like not paying the rent; you end up with no place to live.*

(Gayle Olinekova)

Changing lifestyle

Each of us has a lifestyle that impacts on our health. Naidoo and Wills (2001, p. 280) define lifestyle as:

> *Habits that promote health (eg. regular exercise) or compromise health (eg. smoking). Lifestyles are usually thought of as being individually chosen, but they are also influenced by social factors such as income.*

The health behaviours we adopt in our lifestyle are important indicators in determining morbidity and mortality (Naidoo and Wills, 2001).

Bennett and Murphy (1997) refer to McQueen's (1987) work of the 'holy four' which are associated with disease. The 'holy four' are smoking, alcohol misuse, poor nutrition and low levels of physical activity. Blane *et al* (1998, p. 91) provide examples of the effect of these life course behaviours:

> *An individual whose behaviours include cigarette smoking and high consumption of saturated fats is more likely to be exposed to psychosocial hazards such as multiple environmental stresses and employment conditions which combine high effort with low reward; and also be at greater risk of exposure to occupational hazards, residential damp, local atmospheric pollution and financial constraints on dietary purchases. Conversely, an individual whose behaviours exemplify the medically recommended healthy lifestyle, is more likely to be employed in an occupation which offers autonomy and career prospects, and is less likely to be at the risk of exposure to material hazards because of non-manual work, good quality housing, rural or suburban residence and income.*

As stated above, there are a variety of factors, which impinge on health, such as housing, education, transport, and employment. Education has a strong impact on a person's self-esteem and employment opportunities. It provides a structure to one's life and a perspective of being part of society. In the document *Investing for Health* (Department of Health, Social Services and Public Safety [DHSSP], 2002), education is believed to have a strong impact on how we think about our health, shaping values, beliefs and behaviours as well as key relationships. There is a direct correlation between poverty, poor educational attainment and poor health.

The Health Belief Model is used to predict whether individuals are likely to make changes to their lifestyle by incorporating preventative health behaviours. Naidoo and Wills (2001) provide a good example of this:

> *The health belief model would predict smoking cessation if an individual perceived that she was highly susceptible to lung cancer, that lung cancer was a serious health threat, that the benefits of stopping smoking (for example, more money and less odour) were high and that the costs of such action (for example, potential weight gain or isolation in the peer group) were comparatively low. Furthermore, she is more likely to give up if she is subjected to cues to action that are external, such as a leaflet in the doctor's waiting room, or internal, such as a symptom such as breathlessness perceived (correctly or otherwise) to be related to lung cancer.*
>
> (Naidoo and Wills, 2001, p. 88)

Making changes to one's lifestyle is a complex issue involving lay understandings of disease and its causes, risk and a range of socio-economic factors (Wiles and Kinmonth, 2001). In their qualitative research study, Wiles and Kinmonth (2001) aimed to explore patients' understanding of a heart attack and identify ways of effective secondary prevention strategies. From in-depth interviews with twenty-five patients with myocardial infarction, they found that lay understandings of heart attack were strongly influenced by information from health professionals, the timing of which was important. While motivation for accepting information was high immediately following their heart attack, over time this fell. Noticeably, the amount of information from health professionals reduced over time with the norm being that after the patient's six-week check-up, if there were no complications, patients would be discharged and receive little routine contact from community health professionals. Wiles and Kinmonth advocate that for secondary prevention to be effective, health professionals need to realise that people's understandings and motivations change over time. When engaging in health promotion activities, they should firstly elicit the patient's perceptions of their illness and then integrate these with the appropriate lifestyle changes required.

In their quantitative research study, Song and Lee (2001) found that motivation to make lifestyle changes was improved by an educational programme. The two-day programme involved a multi-disciplinary approach. Day one focused on enhancement of motivation through understanding of an individual's health risks related to their current lifestyle, and making personal goals to change their behaviours. The format of the second day (eight weeks later) was on confirming and maintaining changes in their lifestyles. Through the educational programme individuals were able to improve the patient's perceptions of benefits and barriers to improving their diet and exercise behaviour. However, the education programme did not improve stress management or smoking cessation.

Wyn and Solis (2001) note that doctor-patient discussion about changing lifestyle behaviours is inconsistent. In their paper, which focused on survey data from the Commonwealth Fund 1998 Survey of Women's Health, they report that 60% of women visiting their doctor did not receive any discussion relating to the need to modify their lifestyle behaviours despite the fact that the need was clearly there.

Gabhainn *et al* (1999) conducted a qualitative study using focus group methodology. In total, they recruited seventy-four Irish individuals who were arranged into sixteen groups in the following categories: men and women, blue and white-collar occupations and those under and over forty-five years of age. They found that overall knowledge levels were high with all risk factors associated with cardiovascular disease noted except for lack of exercise. This omission was particularly evident in younger participants in blue-collar groups. They found that respondents were predominantly unmotivated to change due to scepticism about medical advice. Barriers to making lifestyle changes centred on the difficulty of changing routines and habits. Men, particularly older men, were less motivated to change than women. Parmenter (2002) states that people have little motivation to change their diet unless they acknowledge that they have a health concern or illness.

However, it must also be recognised that socio-economic issues affect a healthy lifestyle. An individual's financial capabilities may preclude purchasing healthier foods and a lack of access to a car can create difficulties such as shopping in out-of-town shopping centres or participating in many forms of exercise or sport (Koivusilta *et al*, 1999).

As a means of supporting the health information needs of the population, the Government introduced three additional components in the document *Saving Lives: Our Healthier Nation* (Department of Health [DoH], 1999). These additional components are NHS Direct, first aid skills and the use of patients as experts.

NHS Direct is aimed at empowering people by providing a rapid access to health advice and information via a nurse-led telephone help-line. NHS Direct was launched in 2000, and provides access to health information and professional advice twenty-four hours a day, 365 days a year.

The second initiative was the promotion of teaching young people and others, the basic skills of first aid and resuscitation and thirdly, the support of patient-led support groups. These acknowledge that individuals with chronic and debilitating illnesses are the experts when it comes to coping with their condition. Using patients as experts affords an additional resource in the armoury of factors used to improve health.

To provide some context, mortality rates at all ages are higher in Scotland and Wales than in England. The rates for standardised mortality is 12% higher in Scotland than England for those aged over sixty-five years and 22% higher for those from nought to sixty-five years of age. Scotland and Wales also have higher death rates from lung, breast and cervical cancer than England (Pollock, 1999).

Saving Lives: Our Healthier Nation (DoH, 1999)

This is an action plan through which the Government aims to tackle poor health. The aim is to improve the health of everyone, particularly those who are worst off. The plan is focused on the five major killers in the UK: cancer, coronary heart disease, stroke, accidents and mental illness.

By 2010, by achieving the following targets, it is predicted that some 300,000 untimely and unnecessary deaths will be prevented.

❖ Cancer — to reduce the death rate in people under seventy-five by at least one fifth.

❖ Coronary heart disease (CHD) and stroke — to reduce the death rate in people under seventy-five by at least two fifths.

❖ Accidents — to reduce the death rate by at least one fifth and serious injury by at least a tenth.

❖ Mental illness — to reduce the death rate from suicide and undetermined injury by at least one fifth.

In order to implement the action plan, the Government stated, in the document in 1999, that it would:

- put in more money — £21 billion for the NHS alone to help secure a healthier population
- tackle smoking as the single biggest preventable cause of poor health
- integrate Government and local government to work together in improving health
- stress health improvement as a key role for the NHS
- press for high health standards for all, not just the privileged few (DoH, 1999).

According to Schifrin (2001), less than 7% of the United Kingdom's gross national product is spent on health care compared with 14% in the USA. Scotland's health record remains poor. Some £1.25 billion spent in 1996–97 on incapacity and invalidity benefit in Scotland to people not well enough to work is one measure of the extent of ill health. The life expectancy at birth for both genders in Scotland in 1994 was lower than that in many other industrialised countries. Scotland has the highest mortality rate from coronary heart disease for men and the second highest for women.

The prevalence of CHD among women aged fifty-five to sixty-four in Scotland is almost twice the rate for women in England in the same age group (*Scottish Office, 1998*).

Key points contained within *Saving Lives: Our Healthier Nation* **(DoH, 1999)**

❖ In the forty-six to sixty-five age group, 25% of professional women and 17% of professional men report a limiting long-standing illness, compared to 45% of unskilled women and 48% of unskilled men.

❖ A third of children in the UK live with at least one adult smoker, but among low income families, the figure is 57%.

❖ Nearly one in five working age households has no one in work.

❖ One in five people in Great Britain have persistently low incomes.

❖ In 1996/97, 4.5 million children were being brought up in families with below average income, three times the number twenty years ago.

❖ The life expectancy of a baby boy with parents in the professional or managerial groups is estimated to be about five years more than one born to parents in partly skilled or unskilled occupations.

❖ At the age of twenty-two months, children with parents in the professional or managerial groups who have received higher education are 14% higher up the educational development distribution than those with two parents in partly skilled or unskilled occupations.

❖ Children in receipt of free school meals (about 15% of pupils in England) have lower educational achievement than other children.

❖ In 1997, the rate of unemployment for people with no qualifications was double that for people with five or more GCSE passes at grades A* to C (or the technical equivalent).

❖ A middle-aged man who loses his job doubles his chances of dying in the next five years.

❖ Properties in bad condition are occupied disproportionately by older and single people. People from ethnic minority groups are generally more likely to be poorly housed than white people.

❖ In 1996 there were at least 4.3 million 'fuel poor' householders who need to spend 10% of their income just to keep their homes warm.

❖ Pedestrian fatality rates for children of unskilled parents are five times higher than those of professional parents and are higher for boys than girls.

❖ People in lower socio-economic groups tend to eat less fruit and vegetables and less food that is rich in dietary fibre than other groups. They are also more likely to smoke.

❖ Women are more likely than men to eat wholemeal bread, fruit and vegetables at least once a day and to drink semi-skimmed milk.

❖ People in lower income groups tend to pay more for their food because the physical inaccessibility of large retails outlets, such as out-of-town supermarkets, necessitates expenditure on transport or paying higher prices in small local shops.

❖ In 1996, 11% of women in professional jobs smoked compared to 36% of women in unskilled manual occupations.

❖ Children whose parents smoke are more likely to develop lung illness and other conditions such as glue ear and asthma than children of non-smoking parents.

❖ Teenage girls from poor neighbourhoods are more likely to become pregnant and teenagers account for more than one in ten births in some inner city areas.

❖ The median age at which people first have sex is two years lower among males and females from manual households than those from professional ones.

❖ About half of pregnancies in under sixteens and a third among sixteen to nineteen-year-olds are terminated.

Unemployment and poverty

Poverty is a disease that saps people's energy, dehumanises them and creates a sense of helplessness and loss of control over one's life. Health is a vital asset for the poor. Without health, a person's potential to escape from poverty is weakened due to lost time, labour income and

*the burden of health care costs... Of those who are poor,
70% are female. Children who grow up in poverty are
often permanently damaged due to lack of nourishment
and opportunity.*

(http://www.icn.ch/matterspoverty.html)

Having a sense of control is believed to:

*... mediate associations between socio-economic status
and well-being... and a lack of control is associated with
heightened physiological stress responsivity in... humans,
poor tolerance of pain and worse mental health.*

(Steptoe and Wardle, 2001, p. 659)

Naidoo and Wills (1998, p. 73) state that absolute poverty relates to
the inability to meet the basic biological needs of food, warmth and
shelter, whereas relative poverty means poverty as defined in
relation to the living standards and expectations of contemporary
society. Roach (2000) reports findings from a UNICEF league table of
relative child poverty in which the bottom four places are occupied by
the UK, Italy, USA and Mexico. The report states that to raise
children out of poverty in the UK would cost less than 0.5% of the
gross national product. Kmietowicz (2001) reports that although the
figures of children living in poverty in the UK has fallen by a third
over the last two years, there remain 3 million children living in
poverty and a further 2.4 million experiencing multiple deprivation.
As by way of an example to highlight the long-term effects of childhood poverty, Smith (1999) reports that a boy born to professional or
managerial parents has a five-year longer life expectancy to a boy born
to parents who are in partly or unskilled occupations.

Naidoo and Wills (1998) assert that poverty affects health
through physical, psychological and behavioural dimensions.
Physical effects include the consequence of living in damp, mouldy
and overcrowded conditions. Dyer (2002b) states that people living
in damp housing are up to three times more likely to have asthma
than those in the general population. Behavioural effects include
smoking, drug misuse, poor diet and reduced or no physical exercise.
Psychological effects include feelings of stress, anxiety, depression
and a reduced self-esteem. Weich and Lewis (1998) report that
unemployment and poverty are factors in maintaining episodes of
psychological distress but, in their opinion, they are not the sole
contributors.

Poverty is bad for health in a number of different ways. People who are poor spend less on good food, warm and comfortable housing and are excluded from many activities that others take for granted. They are more likely to be unemployed and unskilled. Children from poor families are more likely to leave school with few or no formal qualifications and to live in insecure and unsafe environments. They are therefore less likely to face their future with hope and self-confidence, to feel in control of their lives and value themselves (DHSSPS, 2002).

Unemployment is the single greatest cause of poverty. Unemployment stigmatises the individual and entails the loss of status, power and self-esteem. Loss of employment causes loss of income, structure and routine to one's life. The former obviously contributes to poverty and the latter to a feeling of aimlessness, alienation and social exclusion (Iphofen and Poland, 1998). Woods and Mitchell (1998) state that women, more than men, are likely to experience poverty, and that 71% of the elderly poor are women. It is estimated that as much as 70% of the world's poor are women and it is argued that this reflects the position of women in society, their unequal situation in the labour market and generally their low status both inside and outside the home (WHO, 1998b).

There is a strong association between unemployment and poor health (Heslop *et al*, 2001).

> *Health inequality is widespread... (it) runs throughout life from before birth through to old age. It exists between social classes, different areas of the country, between males and females, and between people from different ethnic backgrounds.*

> (Heslop *et al*, 2001)

Kunst and Mackenbach (1994) provide a definition of health inequality; namely, the 'differences in the prevalence or incidence of health problems between individual people of higher and lower socio-economic status' (cited by Bull and Hamer, undated).

The poorer you are, the more likely you are to be ill and die younger. Poverty, low wages, occupational stress, unemployment, poor housing, environmental pollution, poor education, limited access to transport and shops, crime and disorder and lack of recreational facilities all have an impact on people's health (DoH, 1999). The extent of the problem is outlined by the following facts from *Our Healthier Nation: Action Report*. Nearly 1:5 households containing working age individuals have no one in work; 1:5 people in the UK have persistently low incomes; a middle-aged man who loses his job doubles his chances of dying in the next five years and in 1996/97, 4.5 million children were brought up in households with below average income which represents three times the number twenty years ago.

Key facts regarding women and poverty

❖ Seventy per cent of the 1.2 billion people living in poverty are female.

❖ Estimates over a twenty-year period found the increase in numbers of poor rural women in forty-one developing countries to be 17% higher than the increase in poor men.

❖ There are twice as many women as men among the world's 900 million illiterates.

❖ Protein-energy malnutrition is significantly higher in women in South Asia, where almost half the world's undernourished reside, half a million women die unnecessarily from pregnancy-related complications each year, the causes of which are exacerbated by issues of poverty and remoteness.

❖ On average, women are paid 30–40% less than men for comparable work.

❖ In developing countries, only a tiny fraction of women hold real economic or political power. In some parts of the world, social roles and cultural norms for poor women may inhibit their willingness or ability to seek health care.

❖ Poverty is a significant factor behind stress and depression in women, with domestic violence a frequent contributing factor.

❖ Poverty is also linked to inadequate access to food and nutrition and the health of older women often reflects the cumulative impact of poor diet.

(Source: WHO, 2000b, c)

The likelihood of unemployment is more evident in the lower social class groups and both within white and ethnic minority groups, women are more likely to be unemployed. This gender difference is particularly pronounced in Pakistanis and Bangladeshis (Cooper, 2002). In general terms, Arber and Khlat (2002) state that women have less power, social status, financial resources, autonomy and independence than men. According to the WHO (2000b), a disproportionate share of the burden of poverty rests on women which in turn undermines their health.

Health inequality

The Government has made the reduction of health inequalities a cornerstone in its health-related policies and requiring locally set initiatives to achieve its aim (Kendall, undated). Kendall cites the WHO in reference to inequality:

> *The term inequality has a moral and ethical dimension. It refers to differences that are unnecessary and avoidable, but, in addition, are also unfair and unjust. So, in order to describe a certain situation as inequitable, the cause has to be examined and judged to be unfair in the context of what is going on in the rest of society... Equity in health implies that ideally everyone should have a fair opportunity to attain their full health potential, and more pragmatically, that no-one should be disadvantaged from achieving this potential if it can be avoided.*

Inequality is described using the Register General's classification of people into initially five and, since 2001, eight occupational categories. Social class I relates to those in professional occupations and social class V relates to those in unskilled manual occupations. The additional three categories reflect changes in the labour market, such as the rising number of those self-employed or long-term unemployed (Naidoo and Wills, 2001). Iphofen and Poland (1998) express the belief that those born into certain social groups will be socialised through education, work, family life, cultural habits and legislation, to expect different life experiences and chances than those born into other social classes. In the UK, the term health inequality refers to the differences between social groups (Marmot, 2001).

Social class differences have been apparent in the UK since the 1840s (Blane *et al*, 1998). A seminal piece of research into health inequalities was the work published in the Black Report (1980;

Townsend, 1988). This report drew attention to the fact that individuals in the more affluent social classes experienced less illness and premature deaths than those in less affluent groups. Subsequent research has confirmed these findings and provided further evidence that children living in deprivation have a greater chance of developing illnesses in adulthood, and that there is a greater predominance of people with poor health among those at the bottom of the social class hierarchy (Cooper, 2002).

Individuals in lower social classes engage in a series of risks, which lead to ill health. According to Koivusilta *et al* (1999), the risk behaviours include: smoking, excessive consumption of alcohol, lack of exercise, poor sleeping patterns, poor diet, coffee drinking and engaging generally in high-risk activities.

Those individuals who experience unemployment, particularly over long periods, are more likely to suffer from both physical and psychological health problems (Fergusson *et al*, 2001; Novo *et al*, 2001; Westerlund *et al*, 2001). Reading and Reynolds (2001) report that the severity of male suicide attempts were directly related to the severity of debt.

Fergusson *et al* (2001) suggest that young people who are unemployed for over six months have a greater incidence of mental health problems, criminal behaviour and substance abuse than their employed counterparts and, indeed, they assert that they are up to eight times more likely to attempt suicide.

Persistent unemployment and poverty leads to social inequalities and a greater risk of health problems (Benzeval and Judge, 2001). Low-income families experience material deprivation through poor diet, and inadequate housing (Stewart-Brown, 2000). A high percentage of those living in poverty are one-parent families. Women who are lone parents are at a greater risk of experiencing depression than couples with children (Reading and Reynolds, 2001). McMunn *et al* (2001) report that in the UK in 1995 there were 1.56 million one-parent families representing 20% of British children. They state that such children are more likely to have behavioural and developmental problems and are at twice the risk of long-term ill effects than children from two-parent families, but they stress that this is due to the effects of poverty rather than the lone parenting. Mayor (2001) points out that women living in poor socio-economic conditions are twenty times more likely to die from problems associated with pregnancy and childbirth than their counterparts in the higher social class groups.

Barrett (2001) reports that minority ethnic groups are more likely to be living in poverty than the rest of the population. Some

35% Chinese, 40% African/Caribbean/Indian and 80% Pakistani and Bangladeshi people have incomes which are 50% of the national average compared to 28% of the white population.

In the UK, social inequalities in health have widened in the last fifty years (Stewart-Brown, 2000) and the *NHS Plan* (DoH, 2000) sets out to reduce the gap by focusing on preventative health measures and working with other agencies to address social, environmental and economic problems.

Key points from the *NHS Plan* (DoH, 2000)

❖ Life expectancy at birth for a boy born into the lowest social class is seventy years compared to seventy-five years in the higher social classes.

❖ Men in the bottom two social classes are three times more likely to die from stroke or coronary heart disease.

❖ Unemployed men have a higher mortality rate, regardless of disease cause, than employed men.

❖ Unemployed women have a higher mortality from coronary heart disease and suicide than employed women.

❖ Men in manual employment are 40% more likely to report long-standing illness than those in non-manual employment.

The *NHS Plan* (2000) sets out three key developments to address the problems associated with health inequalities with a focus more on health improvement rather than a fix and mend philosophy (Hunter, 2001). These developments are to:

• devise national targets
• set up healthy communities aimed at identifying ways of achieving innovation and disseminating good practice
• introduce integrated public health groups across NHS regional and government offices.

The *NHS Plan* (2000) embarked on a mission to improve the health of the population of England by investment and reform. There is a heavy emphasis on prevention and the need to address inequalities. The *NHS Plan* (2000) provides the first national inequalities targets. These include, starting with children under one year, by 2010 to reduce by at least 10% the gap in mortality between manual groups and the population as a whole; and starting with Health Authorities, by 2010, to reduce by at least 10% the gap between the quintile of areas with lowest life expectancy at birth and population as a whole/ (DoH, 2001c).

To achieve this the plan purports to increase and improve the level of primary care in deprived areas, introduce screening programmes for women and children, increase the smoking cessation services and improve the diet of young children by making fruit freely available in schools for four to six-year-olds.

Key points from *Our Healthier Nation: Action Report*

❖ People in lower socio-economic groups tend to eat less fruit, vegetables and other high fibre food than other groups.

❖ People in lower socio-economic groups are more likely to smoke.

❖ People in lower socio-economic groups tend to pay more for their food because of lack of transport to out-of-town supermarkets.

❖ Children of the age of five in the North West Thames region have 59% more tooth decay than those in the South Thames region, and at age twelve the percentage rises to 75%.

❖ In 1996, at least 4.3 million people were fuel poor requiring to spend a minimum of 10% of their income keeping warm.

Policies developed to tackle inequalities are outlined in *Our Healthier Nation: Action Report*:

1. Health improvement programmes which identify and meet local health care needs including inequalities.
2. Primary care groups (PCGs) to design a framework for local service delivery and promoting health improvement.
3. Health action zones (HAZs) to develop local strategies to improve health and health inequalities and build new ways of working together in partnership. There are over twenty-six HAZs in both urban and rural settings catering for thirteen million people.
4. Healthy living centres which were established with £300 million of lottery funding. These centres fund innovative projects, especially

in the most deprived areas. Healthy living centres complement HAZs and local health improvement strategies (Salisbury, 1999).

An additional crucial element of Government policy focuses on the inequalities experienced by individuals from ethnic minorities. The Scottish Executive (2002) states that ethnic minority relates to all subgroups of the population not indigenous to the UK who hold cultural traditions and values derived, at least in part, from their countries of origin. The term 'black' refers to those members of the ethnic minority groups who are differentiated by their skin colour or physical appearance, and may feel some solidarity with one another by reason of past or current experience, but who may also have many different cultural traditions and values.

Lees (2002) refers to the inquiry into inequalities in health, which was chaired by Acheson in 1998. The inquiry reported that people from ethnic minority groups were more likely to report difficulty in gaining access to health care services, particularly those in primary care, and to voice dissatisfaction with the quality of the service that they do receive. Obeid (2001) predicts that by 2005, 50% of the population of Birmingham will be from ethnic minority groups. Another example of the problems associated with communication difficulties and quality of health outcomes is provided by Mayor (2001). Mayor describes research findings which highlight that women from ethnic minority groups are twice as likely to die from causes related to pregnancy and childbirth than white women. Mayor states that the research found that most of the ethnic women spoke no or very poor English and that many of those who died had either missed over four routine appointments or had not 'booked in' until after twenty-four weeks' gestation. These examples, as Obeid asserts, place increased demands on the requirement for multi-lingual health education material, interpreters and link workers. A compounding factor for those living in deprived areas is that despite the indisputable fact that health inequalities exist (Saxena *et al*, 1999; Lazenbatt *et al*, 2000), they often receive poorer health care services and are less likely to use preventative services (Pollock and Vickers, 1998; Smith, 1999).

Researchers have noted that those in employment are more likely to be healthier, offering the following factors as why this might be so. Being in work offers individuals social support (Evans and Steptoe, 2002), and provides a feeling of being in control over one's life (Bailis *et al*, 2001). However, this does not mean that there are no adverse effects on health from being employed. Individuals whose jobs are monotonous, repetitive and lack control are at greater risk of health problems than those who have a high degree of control (Evans and Steptoe, 2002). Women are more likely than men to be in paid work in which they lack control (Karasek and Thoeorell, 1990, cited by Matthews and Power, 2002). Rosenfield (1989) cited by Matthews and Power (2002) found that women experienced more control in their housework role than in paid employment.

Suggested web resources

http://www.hebs.scot.nhs.uk/ Health promotion, Scotland

http://www.doh.gov.uk/healthinequalities The Department of Health's website that sets out policy on health inequalities, national targets and indicators.

http://www.hpe.org.uk/ Health promotion, England

http://www.hpw.wales.gov.uk/ Health promotion, Wales

http://www.jrf.org.uk/ The Joseph Rowntree Foundation provides information relating to community development, health and social inclusion projects. Research includes the developments of key indicators of poverty and social exclusion

http://www.medic8.com. Recommended for finding medical information on the Internet. It is a peer-led medical portal for health professionals. Access is free, no registration is required and no banner advertisements are shown

http://www.nchod.nhs.uk/ The National Centre for Health Outcomes Development provides data and information on measurement too old for public health. It is a key source of information on assessment of health and outcomes of health interventions at a variety of levels

http://www.phs.ik.se/hprin Health promotion research Internet network with links to child and adolescent health promotion

http://www.doh.gov.uk/research/index.net Research and development in the Department of Health and the NHS

http://www.who.dk World Health Organization, Europe

http://www.womens-health.co.uk

References

Arber S, Khlat M (2002) Introduction to social and economic patterning of women's health in a changing world. *Soc Sci Med* **54**: 643–7

Bailis DS, Segall A, Mahon MJ, Chipperfield JG, Dunn EM (2001) Perceived control in relation to socioeconomic and behavioral resources for health. *Soc Sci Med* **52**(11): 1661–76

Barrett S (2001) Improving Access and Quality for Ethnic Minority Women. *Women's Health* **11**(4): 345–54

Beattie A (1991) Knowledge and control in health promotion: a test case for social policy and social theory. In: Gabe J, Calnan M, Bury M, eds. *The Sociology of the Health Service*. Routledge, London: 162–202

Bennett P, Murphy S (1997) *Psychology and Health Promotion*. Open University Press, Aylesbury

Benzeval M, Judge K (2001) Income and health: the time dimension. *Soc Sci Med* **52**: 1424–5

Blane D, Bartley M, Smith GD (1998) Making sense of socio-economic health inequalities. In: Field D, Taylor S, eds. *Sociological Perspectives on Health, Illness and Health Care*. Blackwell Publishing, Oxford: chapter 5

Bull J, Hamer L (undated) *Closing the gap: setting local targets to reduce health inequalities*. Health Development Agency http://www.hda-online.org.uk/research/publications.html (accessed March 2002)

Cooper H (2002) Investigating socio-economic explanations for gender and ethnic inequalities in health. *Soc Sci Med* **54**: 693–706

Department of Health (1999) *Saving Lives: Our Healthier Nation*. DoH, London

Department of Health (2000) *The NHS Plan: A plan for investment, a plan for reform*. CM4818, HMSO, London

Department of Health (2001c) *Priorities and Planning Framework 2002/2003*. DoH, London. http://www.doh.gov.uk/planning2002-2003/index.html (accessed January 2002)

Department of Health, Social Services and Public Safety (2002) *Investing for Health*. http://www.dhsspsni.gov.uk/publications/ (accessed January 2002)

Downie RS, Tannahill C, Tannahill A (1996) *Health Promotion: Models and values*. 2nd edn. Oxford University Press, Oxford

Dyer O (2002b) More than two million homes are cold enough to cause ill health, Shelter says. *Br Med J* **324**: 634

Evans O, Steptoe A (2002) The contribution of gender-role orientation, work factors and home stressors to psychological well-being and sickness absence in male- and female-dominated occupational groups. *Soc Sci Med* **54**: 481–92

Eweles L, Simnett I (1999) *Promoting Health: A Practical Guide*. 4th edn. Baillière Tindall, London

Fergusson DM, Horwood J, Woodward LJ (2001) Unemployment and psychosocial adjustment in young adults: causation or selection? *Soc Sci Med* **53**: 305–20

Gabhainn SN, Kelleher CC, Naughton AM, Carter F, Flanagan M, McGrath MJ (1999) Socio-demographic variations in perspectives on cardiovascular disease and associated risk factors. *Health Educ Res* **14**(5): 619–28

Heslop P, Smith GD, Macleod J, Hart C (2001) The socioeconomic position of employed women, risk factors and mortality. *Soc Sci Med* **53**(4): 477–85

Hunter DJ (2001) The NHS Plan: a new direction for English public health? *Crit Public Health* **11**(1): 75–81

Iphofen R, Poland F (1998) *Sociology in Practice for Health Care Professionals*. Macmillan, Basingstoke

Karasek RA, Theorell T (1990) *Healthy Work*. Basic Books, New York

Kawachi I, Kennedy B (1997) Socio-economic determinants of health: health and social cohesion: why care about income equality? *Br Med J* **314**: 1037

Kendall L (undated) *Local Inequalities Targets*. King's Fund, London

Kendall S, Lask S (1997) *Promoting the Health of the Nation*. Churchill-Livingstone, Edinburgh

Kmietowicz Z (2001) UK child poverty falls by a third. *Br Med J* **322**: 510

Koivusilta LK, Rimpela AH, Rimpela MK (1999) Health-related lifestyle in adolescence — origin of social class differences in health? *Health Educ Res* **14**(3): 339–55

Kunst A, Mackenbach J (1994) *Measuring Socio-economic Inequalities in Health*. WHO (unpublished monograph), Geneva

Lazenbatt A, Orr J, Bradley M, McWhirter L, Chambers M (2000) Tackling inequalities in health and social wellbeing: Evidence of 'good practice' by nurses, midwives and health visitors. *Int J Nurs Practice* 6: 76–88

Lees C (2002) Are district nurses meeting the needs of ethnic minorities? JCN January. http://www.jcn.co.uk/printFriend.asp?ArticleID=431 (accessed March 2002)

Liimatainen L, Poskiparta M, Sjogren A, Kettunen T, Karhila P (2001) Investigating student nurses' constructions of health promotion in nursing education. *Health Educ Res* 16(1): 33–48

Marmot M (2001) Economic and social determinants of disease. *Bull World Health Organ* 79(10): 988–9

Matthews S, Power C (2002) Socio-economic gradients in psychological distress: a focus on women, social roles and work-home characteristics. *Soc Sci Med* 54: 799–810

Mayor S (2001) Poorest women 20 times more likely to die in childbirth. *Br Med J* 323: 1324

McMunn AM, Nazroo JY, Marmot MG, Boreham R, Goodman R (2001) Children's emotional and behavioural well-being and family environment: findings from the Health Survey for England. *Soc Sci Med* 53: 423–40

McQueen D (1987) *Research in Health Behaviour, Health Promotion and Public Health.* Working paper. Research Unit in Health and Behavioural Change, cited in Bennet and Murphy (1997), Edinburgh

Naidoo J, Wills J (1998) *Practising Health Promotion: Dilemmas and challenges.* Baillière Tindall, London

Naidoo J, Wills J (2001) *Health Studies: An Introduction.* Palgrave, Hampshire

Novo M, Hammarstrom A, Janlert U (2001) Do high levels of unemployment influence the health of those who are not unemployed? A gendered comparison of young men and women during boom and recession. *Soc Sci Med* 53: 293–303

Obeid A (2001) Increasing access to healthcare. *JCN Online* 15(9) http://www.jcn.co.uk (accessed March 2002)

Parmenter K (2002) Changes in nutrition knowledge and dietary behaviour. *Health Educ* 102(1): 23–9

Pollock AM (1999) Devolution and health: challenges for Scotland and Wales. *Br Med J* 318: 1195–7

Pollock AM, Vickers N (1998) Deprivation and emergency admissions for cancers of colorectum, lung and breast in south east England: ecological study. *Br Med J* 317: 245–52

Reading R, Reynolds S (2001) Debt, social disadvantage and maternal depression. *Soc Sci Med* 53(4): 441–53

Roach JO (2000) One in six children live in relative poverty. *Br Med J* 320: 1621

Rosenfield S (1989) The effect of women's employment: Personal control and sex differences in mental health. *J Health Soc Behav* 30: 77–91

Salisbury C (1999) Healthy living centres. *Br Med J* 319: 1384–5

Saxena S, Majeed A, Jones M (1999) Socioeconomic differences in childhood consultation rates in general practice in England and Wales: prospective cohort study. *Br Med J* 318: 642–6

Schifrin E (2001) An overview of Women's Health Issues in the United States and United Kingdom. *Women's Health Issues* 11(4): 261–81

Scottish Executive (2002) *Fair for All.* Scottish Executive, Edinburgh

Scottish Office (1998) *Working Together for a Healthier Scotland.* Department of Health, Scottish Office

Smith R (1999) Eradicating child poverty. *Br Med J* 319: 203

Song R, Lee H (2001) Managing health habits for myocardial infarction (MI) patients. *Int J Nurs Stud* **38**: 375–80

Steptoe A, Wardle J (2001) Locus of control and health behaviour revisited: A multivariate analysis of young adults from 18 countries. *Br J Psychol* **92**: 659–72

Stewart-Brown S (2000) What causes social inequalities: why is this question taboo? *Crit Public Health* **10**(2): 233–42

Tannahill A (1985) What is health promotion? *Health Educ J* **44**: 167–8

Tones K (1991) Health promotion, empowerment and the psychology of control. *J Institute of Health Education* **29**(19): 17–25

Tones K (2002) Reveille for Radicals! The paramount purpose of health education? *Health Educ Res* **17**(1): 1–5

Tones K, Tilford S (2001) *Health Promotion: Effectiveness, Efficiency and Equity*. Nelson Thornes, London

Townsend P, Davidson N, Whitehead M (1988) *Inequalities in Health: The Black Report/The Health Divide*. Penguin, London

Walker L (2000) Educating the Educators. *JCN Online* **14**(16) http://www.jcn.co.uk (accessed March 2002)

Weich S, Lewis G (1998) Poverty, unemployment, and common mental disorders: population based cohort study. *Br Med J* **317**: 115–9

Westerlund H, Theorell T, Bergstrom A (2001) Psychophysiological effects of temporary alternative employment. *Soc Sci Med* **52**: 405–15

World Health Organization (1986) *Ottawa Charter for Health Promotion*. WHO, Geneva

World Health Organization (1998a) *Health Promotion Glossary*. WHO, Geneva

World Health Organization (1998b) *Gender and Health: Technical paper*. WHO, Geneva

World Health Organization (2000b) *Gender, Health and Poverty. Fact sheet No. 251*. WHO, Geneva

World Health Organization (2000c) *Women, Ageing and Health. Fact sheet No. 252*. WHO, Geneva

Wiles R, Kinmonth A (2001) Patients' understandings of heart attacks: implications for prevention of recurrence. *Patient Educ Counselling* **44**: 161–9

Woods MF, Mitchell ES (1997) Preventative Health Issues: The perimenopausal to mature years (45–64). In: Allen KM, Phillips JM, eds. *Women's Health: Across the lifespan*. Lippincott, Philadelphia

Wyn R, Solis B (2001) Women's health issues across the lifespan. *Women's Health Issues* **11**(3): 148–59

2

Maintaining a healthy heart and lungs

Introduction

This chapter addresses the health issues related to maintaining a healthy cardiovascular and respiratory system. A major factor discussed is the effect cigarette smoking has on both systems. Discussion revolves around the prevalence of smoking among women and young people, reasons why individuals commence smoking and factors that facilitate and inhibit smoking cessation.

Cardiovascular disease

Cardiovascular disease is defined as including coronary heart disease (CHD), stroke, peripheral vascular disease and heart failure (Wallis *et al*, 2000). Two of the major cardiovascular diseases (CVDs) are coronary heart disease and stroke. According to the British Heart Foundation (BHF) (2002) there are over 235,000 deaths a year attributable to CVD, which accounts for four out of ten of all deaths. Indeed, CVD is also one of the main causes of premature death (45,000 in 2000); 36% of premature deaths in men and 28% in women. Deaths from CVD are mostly due to coronary heart disease, while a quarter are attributed to stroke. Pakistani and Bangladeshi people have considerably higher rates of coronary heart disease than white people (Smith *et al*, 2000).

Coronary heart disease (CHD)

Coronary heart disease is defined as a fatal or non-fatal myocardial infarction plus incident angina (Wallis *et al*, 2000). In the foreword to the Coronary Heart Disease/Stroke Taskforce Report (2001) the chief medical officer wrote when referring to coronary heart disease and stroke as major causes of ill health and death, ' ... the leading causes of death are actually smoking, unhealthy diets, excess alcohol and too little exercise'. Scotland's death rate from coronary heart disease and stroke remains the second highest in western Europe.

Key facts

* ❖ One in six women die from CHD.
* ❖ Twenty-eight per cent of premature deaths in women are due to CVD.
* ❖ Premature death rate from stroke is double in manual workers than those in non-manual occupations.
* ❖ It is estimated that there are about 158,000 new cases of women suffering from angina each year.
* ❖ It is estimated that there are 30,000 new cases of heart failure in women each year.
* ❖ British Heart Foundation (2002) estimates that there are about 1.2 million women in the UK who have coronary heart disease.
* ❖ Scotland has one of the highest death rates from coronary heart disease world-wide. There are approximately half a million people in Scotland with coronary heart disease and it accounts for 12,000 deaths per year.

Coronary heart disease is one of the leading causes of death in the industrialised world (Barnard and Inkeles, 1999; Wiles and Kinmouth, 2001) and according to Schifrin (2001) it is the principal causes of death in the United States and the United Kingdom. The mortality rates within the United Kingdom are higher than many other European countries with one in four deaths being attributed to coronary heart disease (Schifrin, 2001).

In 1996, there were 13,650 (24.1%) deaths caused by coronary heart disease in Scotland (Scottish Executive [SE], 2001). In the same year, there were 15,175 (25%) deaths attributed to cancer. The economic cost of coronary heart disease to the UK is reported to be about £10,000 million a year. This can be contrasted to 1% of that figure which is spent on prevention of the disease (BHF, 2002).

As with many diseases, there is clear evidence of an increasing incidence of coronary heart disease in deprived areas. In Scotland, individuals living in the most deprived areas are two and a half times more at risk from dying from coronary heart disease than those in the least deprived areas (Scottish Executive, 2001).

Every year, approximately 1.5 million people in the UK are diagnosed with one of the commonest symptoms of coronary heart disease; angina. Furthermore, some 270,000 people in the United Kingdom suffer a myocardial infarction (heart attack) and about 30% of these individuals die before reaching hospital. There appears to be some regional differences within the United Kingdom. Deaths from coronary heart disease are higher in Scotland, Ireland and Northern England than elsewhere in the UK. Gabhainn *et al* (1999) assert that the rates of coronary heart disease are particularly high in both parts of Ireland. Tod *et al* (2001) state that compared to death rates from coronary heart disease in England and Wales, Barnsley, Rotherham and Doncaster are among the highest (Tod *et al*, 2001). The premature death rate for men living in Scotland is over 50% higher than their counterparts in East Anglia and 80% higher for women (BHF, 2002).

In 1992 mortality targets for coronary heart disease were set to reduce the death rate in people aged 65–74 by at least 30% (from 899 per 100,000) in 1990 to no more than 629 per 100,000 by the year 2000 (DoH, 1992). The mortality from acute myocardial infarction in men under sixty-five years of age remains between two and three times higher in the most deprived areas. Much of this difference can be explained by the higher rates of cigarette smoking in these deprived areas (Scottish Executive, 2001).

The incidence of coronary heart disease and the associated mortality and morbidity rises with age. The risk of dying from coronary heart disease almost doubles with each decade increase in age (Scottish Executive, 2001). There is also a gender difference (Pocock *et al*, 2001). The incidence in women under fifty-five years of age is one third of that in men. By the time women reach seventy-five years of age, the incidence is equal to that of men. The difference is thought to be due to the protective effect of oestrogen (Schifrin, 2001). It is postulated that oestrogen affects serum lipids and the vascular wall, particularly the inner lining or endothelium, thereby reducing the development of coronary heart disease (Schifrin, 2001). Barnard and Inkeles (1999) note that post-menopausal women who take hormone replacement therapy (HRT) are at a reduced risk for coronary heart disease and stroke. Rousseau (2001) offers the figure of a 40–50% reduction in the risk of coronary heart disease by using hormone replacement therapy.

In the United Kingdom, the mortality rates are falling more slowly in women than in men. There is evidence to suggest that women delay seeking help for symptoms related to coronary heart disease. Van Tiel *et al* (1998) state that women's complaints are less well recognised by doctors as the first signs of coronary heart disease and when they are recognised they are often believed to be less serious. Both genders have a tendency to think that coronary heart disease is a male disease. In their study, Van Tiel *et al* (1998) found that men did not perceive themselves at a higher risk than women, which is contrary to findings from previous research studies. They also found that women tended to delay for longer prior to contacting their general practitioner (GP) than men. Where women did not connect their symptoms with heart disease, the delay was even longer. Holliday *et al* (2000) reinforced the latter finding.

Schifrin (2001) reports a study, which demonstrated that a third of women died within one month of having a myocardial infarction (MI), compared to one sixth of men. Lee (1998) and Hine (2001) suggest that this may be due to women receiving less effective care than men. Lee (1998) notes that although the incidence of coronary heart disease is lower in women than in men, the mortality rates and long-term disability are higher in women than in men. Hine (2001) asserts that women with chronic angina are less likely to receive surgical treatment. Furthermore, those who have suffered a myocardial infarction are less likely to receive thrombolysis or be admitted to a coronary care unit and Hine offers these as reasons why women do worse than men in terms of outcome.

Brink *et al* (2002) report that the first acute episode of myocardial infarction is more likely to be fatal in women than in men as women who develop a myocardial infarction usually do so at an older age than males. Duvernoy and Eagle (2001) assert that women who have suffered a myocardial infarction tend to be older and sicker than their male counterparts and have a poorer prognosis.

The 'National Framework for Coronary Heart Disease' sets a target for GPs and other primary healthcare professionals to identify all people on their lists who have established coronary heart disease and offer them comprehensive advice and appropriate treatment to reduce the risks (Moher *et al*, 2001). It is therefore a government priority to prevent coronary heart disease (CHD framework guidance).

Employment and social class also impinges on the incidence rates of coronary heart disease. Women in manual labour social groups have four times the incidence of the disease than their counterparts in the higher social classes and this gap is widening (Schifrin, 2001). Women under the age of sixty-five experiencing socio-economic deprivation have a two-fold increase in the chance of dying before reaching hospital and are 20% more likely to die within the first month post myocardial infarction (MacIntyre *et al*, 2001).

In the United Kingdom, there are differences in incidence of coronary heart disease according to ethnicity. Women who were born in the Indian sub-continent have a 43% higher death rate from coronary heart disease compared to the country as a whole (Schifrin, 2001). The death rate from coronary heart disease in first generation South Asians (Indians, Bangladeshis, Pakistanis and Sri Lankans) in the age-group twenty to sixty-nine is 50% higher than the average in England and Wales (Barrett, 2001).

Barrett (2001) offers the lack of sensitivity to the healthcare needs of black and minority ethnic groups as an explanation. She believes that the experience of navigating one's way through the NHS is one full of anxiety for those whose first language is not English and, as a result, these individuals do not feel able to discuss all their health problems. She notes, however, that NHS Direct is going some way to address this issue by providing information in thirty different languages.

A significant preventable component in coronary heart disease can be achieved through environmental and lifestyle modification (Gabhainn *et al*, 1999). Moher *et al* (2001) report that the national service framework for coronary heart disease set a target for GPs and primary care teams in England to identify all people with coronary heart disease and offer them comprehensive advice and appropriate treatment to reduce their risks.

It is generally accepted that socio-economic factors impinge directly on incidence of coronary heart disease (MacIntyre *et al*, 2001). It is also accepted that individuals from more deprived areas have low expectations, which may mean that they are less likely to seek help from their GP early in the disease process and they are less likely to be assertive in seeking investigations. Local health care co-operatives (LHCCs) are charged with developing innovative ways of encouraging individuals who have symptoms of coronary heart disease to consult their GP earlier in the progression of the disease (Scottish Executive, 2001). At a local level in Scotland, the following initiatives are in place to help prevent coronary heart disease:

• GP exercise referral schemes
• health board support for community food initiatives, for example, food co-operatives and development of cooking skills, breakfast clubs providing a nutritious start to the day for the children who attend

- encouraging children to become more physically active
- smoking cessation initiatives (Scottish Executive, 2001).

Smoking

Tobacco was introduced to Europe from the New World at the end of the fifteenth century. Amos and Haglund (2000) present a very interesting history of smoking and women. They describe Danish painters using tobacco as a means to portray human folly and women in their paintings were either whores or prostitutes. In the 1850s women did not smoke or, if they did, it was never acknowledged. In the nineteenth century women smokers were generally perceived to be 'fallen' women with smoking being seen as the occupational symbol of prostitution. Amos and Haglund report incidences of women being arrested in the early 1900s for smoking in public. There was a clear stigma associated with women who smoked.

Amos and Haglund (2000) state it was only with the introduction of mass-produced cigarettes that smoking became socially acceptable. They assert that this was due not only to the change in status of women in the last fifty years, but due to the promotion of smoking by the tobacco industry as a symbol of emancipation, liberation and power. Smoking rapidly spread throughout the nineteenth century and was thought to have medicinal value. It was not until the twentieth century that smoking became a mass habit and it was not until the Second World War that the dangers of smoking were firmly established (Action on Smoking and Health [ASH], 2001b).

Currently, there are about 13 million adults who smoke in the United Kingdom. Tobacco smoke contains over 4,000 chemical compounds, which are present either as gases or as tiny particles. The following table from ASH (2001b) (*Table 2.1*) and information from NHS Direct outlines the dangers of just three of these compounds.

Table 2.1: Dangers of three chemical compounds	
Nicotine	This is what is addictive. It stimulates the central nervous system, increasing the heart rate and blood pressure. In large quantities nicotine is extremely poisonous.
Tar	Brown and treacly in appearance, tar consists of tiny particles and is formed when tobacco smoke condenses. Tar is deposited in the lungs and respiratory system and gradually absorbed. It is a mixture of many different chemicals, including: formaldehyde, arsenic, cyanide, benzo(a)pyrene, benzene, toluene, acrolein. Condensed tar can stain smokers' fingers and teeth. Benzene is a known carcinogen and is associated with leukaemia. Formaldehyde is a highly poisonous, colourless liquid used to preserve dead bodies. It is known to cause cancer, respiratory, skin and gastro-intestinal problems.
Carbon monoxide	This is a poisonous gas also found in car exhaust fumes. It binds to haemoglobin in the bloodstream more easily than oxygen, thus making the blood carry up to 15% less oxygen around the body.

(Source: ASH, 2001b)

As can be seen from above, tobacco is a dangerous product and if it were being introduced today it would undoubtedly be illegal.

Extent of the problem

It is estimated that half a billion of today's world population will be killed by the effects of tobacco and 50% of these deaths will occur in middle-age, thereby losing on average twenty years or more of life (Meyrick, 2001).

Professor Richard Peto from the Imperial Cancer Research Fund claims that even with no increase in the rate of cigarette smoking in the UK, some one billion people will die from tobacco-related deaths in the twenty-first century. He compares this to the figure of 100,000 million in the twentieth century. If adult smokers were to stop smoking over the next twenty years, the effect would be one-third reduction in tobacco-related deaths in 2020 (http://www.health-secure.net, accessed October 2002).

In the United Kingdom, it is estimated that health-related behaviours such as smoking, diet and exercise, account for one third of the socio-economic variations in mortality. Over the last two decades, the smoking cessation rates in the UK have reduced in the more economically advantaged groups, however, this is not reflected in the poorer groups in society.

Key facts

❖ Smoking has more than fifty ways of making life a misery through illness and more than twenty ways of killing you.

❖ About 90% of cases of peripheral vascular disease which lead to amputation of one or both legs are caused by smoking — about 2000 amputations a year in the UK.

❖ Smoking kills over 120,000 people in the UK every year. Deaths caused by smoking are six times higher than all the deaths arising from road traffic accidents, poisoning and overdose, accidental deaths, murder and manslaughter, suicide and HIV infection in the UK during 1998.

❖ Risk of lung cancer increases approximately in proportion to the duration of smoking: smoking twenty cigarettes a day for forty years is eight times more hazardous than smoking forty cigarettes a day for twenty years.

❖ People in poorer social classes are more likely to die early due a number of factors. Among men, the dominant factor is smoking which accounts for over 50% of the difference in premature death between the social classes.

❖ In social class I about 14% of women smoke. In social class V, about 33% of women smoke.

❖ Smoking twenty cigarettes a day costs £950 per year using smuggled cigarettes and £1,600 using top brands.

❖ Households in the lowest tenth of income, spend six times as much of their income on tobacco as households in the highest tenth.

❖ Among those living in greatest hardship, smoking rates are 70%.

❖ There is evidence that a smoker's level of nicotine dependence increases systematically with deprivation. Poorer smokers achieve higher intakes of nicotine both by choosing to smoke more cigarettes and by smoking each cigarette more intensively. Since nicotine dependence is an important determinant of ease of quitting, this suggests one reason for the lower rates of cessation in those who are more disadvantaged.

❖ Treating smoking-related illnesses costs the NHS £1.7 billion every year.

(Source: ASH, 2001a)

Smoking has been identified as the primary cause of the health gap between the rich and the poor. Some 70% of people in the most deprived areas of the UK smoke, and around 90% of those who are homeless and sleep rough smoke (Richardson and Crosier, undated). Alan Milburn, Secretary of State for Health stated in the Health Development Agency (HDA) (undated) document entitled *Smoking and Health Inequalities*:

> *Smoking is the principal cause of the inequalities in death rates between the rich and the poor. Put simply, smoking is a public health disaster.*

There is a social class gradient in the prevalence of smoking as can be seen in *Table 2.2*.

Table 2.2: Prevalence of smoking in classes I and V

	Social class I: % of smokers	Social class V: % of smokers
Men	15%	45%
Women	14%	33%

(Source: Richardson and Crosier, undated)

However, Richardson and Crosier (undated) state that these figures mask the high levels of smokers in deprived areas in the UK. There is about a 70% smoking prevalence in the most deprived groups which rises to 90% in those who are homeless and sleeping rough.

There seems to be a regional difference with both adults and teenagers in Scotland and Northern Ireland smoking more than those in England and Wales. In England, smoking rates tend to be higher in the North. Manual workers tend to smoke more than non-manual workers. The British Nutrition Foundation (BNF) (2002) report that 31% of women in manual occupations smoked compared to 21% in non-manual occupations.

Generally, women in ethnic groups have low smoking rates (8% or less). In England and Wales there is a higher incidence of Bangladeshi and Caribbean men smoking than their white counterparts. Few Bangladeshi women smoke (Payne, 2001a). Smith *et al* (2000, p. 399) suggest that religion may have an influence on rates of smoking in ethnic groups since, 'religious limits are placed on smoking among Sikhs... absence of a Muslim prohibition on smoking, although there is a general expectation of restraint for women.'

Smoking prevalence among children and young people

The prevalence of smoking, especially in young women, is expected to continue to rise (Bastian *et al*, 2001). Meyrick (2001) states that young women in developed countries and people of both genders in developing countries continue to smoke reflecting a prevalence rate which is unacceptably high.

The prevalence of females who smoke cigarettes in the UK in 1998 was 26%. Again in 1998, it was estimated that 11% of girls aged eleven to fifteen years were regular smokers, with regular being defined as smoking a minimum of one cigarette per week. This is to be contrasted with increasing rates of smoking in teenage girls, which peaked in 1996. Female adolescents who have low self-esteem are between two and four times more likely to smoke than their counterparts who have a high self-esteem (Oxley, 2001). Oxley (2001) defines self-esteem as the judgements that individuals make about themselves and how they feel about themselves. Coleman and Hendry (1999) state that those with higher self-esteem are more likely to be able to resist peer pressure and less likely to be involved in deviant behaviours such as drug or alcohol misuse.

> *In terms of self-esteem, there is a general agreement that this variable has a powerful influence on adjustment across a wide range of domains. Educational achievement, social relationships, mental health, the ability to deal with stress are all affected by self-esteem.*

(Coleman and Hendry, 1999, p. 70)

Smoking prevalence in young people is an increasing concern. According to ASH (2001b), three out of four children are aware of cigarettes before they reach the age of five whether the parents are smokers or not. By the age of eleven, around 33% of children, and by sixteen, about 66% of children, have experimented with smoking.

The Cancer Working Group (1999) reports that in 1988 one in five teenage girls smoked, but today the ratio is one in three. They state that children as young as eight are smoking and that smokers' life expectancy is estimated to be sixteen years shorter than non-smokers. Spear and Kulbok (2001) report that young people are more likely to start smoking if one or both their parents smoke and that males are more influenced by their friends than by their parents.

Facts on young people and smoking

❖ In the UK, about 450 children start smoking every day.

❖ Approximately 12% of Scottish school children between the ages of twelve and fifteen smoke.

❖ Children are three times as likely to smoke if both their parents smoke.

❖ Children who smoke are between two and six times more susceptible to coughs and increased phlegm, wheeziness and dyspnoea.

❖ Children who smoke are three times more likely to have time off school.

❖ Adolescents from lower socio-economic backgrounds are more likely to smoke every day.

❖ The earlier children become regular smokers and persist in the habit as adults, the greater the risk of dying prematurely.

❖ A recent US study found that smoking during teenage years causes permanent genetic changes in the lungs and increases the risk of lung cancer, even if the smoker subsequently stops.

❖ Children are more susceptible to the effects of passive smoking — those whose parents smoke are estimated to be receiving a nicotine equivalent of smoking eighty cigarettes a year.

❖ Children who experiment with cigarettes quickly become addicted to nicotine in tobacco. Thirty-three per cent of children who smoke one or more cigarettes a week light up their first cigarette within thirty minutes of waking and one in twelve light up within the first five minutes.

❖ Approximately 10% of teenagers aged eleven to fifteen are regular smokers and there has been little change over the past twelve years (Coleman and Hendry, 1999).

❖ Fifty-eight per cent of regular smokers, aged between eleven and fifteen, state that they would find it difficult to give up smoking for a week and 72% thought it would be difficult to give up altogether.

❖ Girls are more likely to smoke than boys.

❖ The younger a person is when they start smoking, the greater the risk of developing lung cancer.

❖ For every 1000 twenty-year-old smokers, it is estimated that one will be murdered, six will die in road traffic accidents, but 250 will die in middle age from smoking and another 250 will die from smoking in older age.

According to a UK Health Authority survey, 24% of girls between fifteen and sixteen smoked on a daily basis compared with 15% of boys. There are certain general characteristics (listed below) associated with teenagers who smoke. They:

- have family members and friends who smoke
- are more likely to come from single parent families
- may have low self-esteem, less confidence and more anxiety
- have poor educational aspirations
- spend their leisure time either in part-time jobs or 'hanging around' (Coleman and Hendry, 1999).

Why do children and young people smoke? There are complex reasons why they take up smoking but there is one consistent factor cited in the literature: the influence of peers and significant others, such as parents and siblings.

There is also evidence that tobacco advertising deliberately designed to appeal to young people is associated with an increased uptake (NHS Centre for Reviews and Dissemination [NHS CRD], 1999). There is also a socio-economic aspect to consider. Children from less advantaged social backgrounds are more likely to start smoking than children from more affluent backgrounds. By the time these children reach their thirties, 50% of the more advantaged children who started smoking have stopped, while 75% of those who were children from less advantaged groups have continued smoking (Richardson and Crosier, undated).

It is becoming increasingly clear that adolescents start smoking for predominately cultural reasons. They are likely to commence smoking in response to social influences of family, friends and others whom they admire. Sargent *et al* (2001) conducted a cross-sectional survey of 4919 American school children in the nine to fifteen age group and observed the rate of smoking in 601 films. They found that there was a strong direct and independent association between higher exposure to tobacco use in films and smoking in adolescents. They estimated that over a year a typical teenager will watch 150 films, exposing themselves to over 800 depictions of smoking. Sargent *et al* assert that by seeing just one film with their favourite film star smoking can be sufficient to affect their attitude to smoking. According to McCool *et al* (2001) tobacco use in films in the last decade has increased. They believe the way in which smoking is portrayed in films may cause smoking to be seen as normal and therefore a credible (and acceptable) response to real life stress and emotional events.

Moffat and Johnson (2001) report that in a large sample of teenage girls from Canada and the UK, smoking was found to be associated with concerns regarding body weight and shape. They found that girls were more likely to smoke to relieve symptoms of depression and continue to smoke to relieve or avoid withdrawal symptoms. They also found some evidence to suggest that teenagers want to stop smoking but are hampered by addiction.

There are two levels of addiction; physical and mental. Physical addiction is associated with the physical withdrawal symptoms when someone first stops or reduces taking tobacco, drugs or alcohol. Mental addiction is associated with cravings and people experience anxiety, depression, disrupted sleep and poor concentration making their life difficult to manage (Mind out for Mental Health, 2002).

Moffat and Johnston (2001) cite Flay's (1993) five-stage model of teenage smoking.

Stage 1. Motivation
Stage 2. Initial trying
Stage 3. Experimentation
Stage 4. Regular use
Stage 5. Nicotine dependence

Mofatt and Johnson (2001) suggest that the estimated time from stage 2 to stage 4 takes two years. The earlier the child begins to smoke, the more likely it is that they will continue to smoke and smoke heavily.

Smoking is viewed by teenagers as a rite of passage into adulthood and that genetic and environmental factors are proposed as significant reasons for starting smoking and reinforcing its continuance (Lawn *et al*, 2002; Rugkasa *et al*, 2001). Meyrick (2001) reports that in the USA it is estimated that 3000 adolescents start smoking every day. Adolescent smokers are at risk of becoming addicted to nicotine by their twenties. Ninety-one per cent of adult smokers started smoking in their adolescence (Meyrick, 2001; Rugkasa *et al*, 2001). Paavola *et al* (2001) declare that the continuity in smoking from teenage years into adulthood is strongly related to the extent to which teenagers regularly smoked. They state that once young people have become weekly smokers they are unlikely to give up.

In 2000, Charlton and Bates added to the complex factors that are believed to contribute to young people smoking. They put forward a theory that the reason why there has been a slight decline in smoking in young people since 1996, is the advent of mobile phones. According to Charlton and Bates, owning a mobile phone offers young people an instant adult style, individuality, sociability, rebellion, peer group bonding and adult aspiration. Furthermore, marketing of mobile phones focuses on promoting one's self-image and adult aspiration, the very qualities that some young people commence smoking to gain. It is certainly an interesting theory but as yet there is no empirical evidence to support it.

Smoking and health-related diseases

Health-related diseases caused as a result of smoking include coronary heart disease, stroke, lung cancer and other lung-related illnesses, and bladder cancer. These form the main reasons why smoking cessation is promoted.

Coronary heart disease

Smoking kills more than thirteen people every hour in every day. Someone who has never smoked is 60% less likely than someone who has smoked to develop coronary heart disease and is 30% less likely to have a stroke. Deciding not to smoke is equivalent to choosing life against chronic ill-health and premature death (DoH, 1999).

Cigarette smoking increases the risk of developing coronary heart disease. The impact of smoking is more noticeable in women and at younger ages (Pocock *et al*, 2001). It is estimated that about 17% of female deaths from coronary heart disease are due to cigarette smoking. Passive smoking is also a risk factor for coronary heart disease. Josefson (2001) reports that even transient, short-term exposure to environmental smoke significantly reduces coronary blood flow in healthy young non-smokers. The American Lung Association estimates that between 35,000 to 50,000 deaths per year are attributable to passive smoking.

Hypertension

Not surprisingly, hypertension is associated with a risk of coronary heart disease. People with hypertension are three times more likely to develop coronary heart disease and stroke and are twice as likely to die from these diseases than those who have normal blood pressure. The higher the blood pressure, the higher the risk (DoH, 2001a).

Primary risk factors for the development of hypertension are advancing age, excess body weight, excessive salt intake, high alcohol consumption, family history and physical inactivity (Garber, 1997).

The British Heart Foundation (2002) report that in England, 33% of women are hypertensive (systolic of 140mmHg or over and a diastolic of 90mmHg or over). The prevalence of hypertension increases with age. An example provided by the British Heart Foundation is that one in six women in the age group sixteen to twenty-four are hypertensive and this rises to 50% in the fifty-five to sixty-four age group and 75% in the over seventy-fives. Pakistani and Black Caribbean women and Chinese women are about 25% more likely to be hypertensive than women in the general population. There is little difference in the prevalence of hypertension among the social classes although it is noted that in women, as their income increases, so does the prevalence of high blood pressure (DoH, 2001a).

The chief medical officer for the Department of Health reports that 37% of strokes could be prevented if hypertension was treated appropriately (DoH, 2001a). Hypertension can be treated by lifestyle changes such as reducing salt intake, increasing consumption of fruit and vegetables, reducing overweight or obesity and increasing physical activity. In the UK, 75% of our salt intake comes from the consumption of processed foods and so the DoH is working with the food industry to reduce this (DoH, 2001a). The DoH priorities and planning framework for 2002/2003 (DoH, 2001b) states that one of the *NHS Plan's* objectives is, by 2010, to reduce deaths from coronary heart disease by 40% in people under seventy-five by meeting the coronary heart disease NSF standards, aiming to improve the health of the worst off in particular. Building on achievements in 2001, the action for 2002/2003 support the roll out of action on a healthy diet, particularly targeting deprived areas, including the planned fifty new Five-a-Day community initiatives and the expansion of the school fruit scheme to cover 600,000 children.

Sacks *et al* (2001) report on their research study that introduced the DASH diet. The DASH diet stands for dietary approaches to stop hypertension. They found that the DASH diet, which emphasises fruit, vegetables, low-fat dairy foods and whole grain products, poultry, fish and nuts and contains reduced amounts of red meat, fats and sugar, lowers blood pressure. Furthermore, combining a reduced salt intake with the DASH diet produced greater reductions in blood pressure.

The DoH (1999) set out actions for reducing the risk of coronary heart disease or stroke. These are as follows:

❖ Reduce the death rate in people under seventy-five from coronary heart disease or stroke by at least two-fifths.

❖ Major changes in diet, particularly among the worst off, with increased consumption of such foods as fruit, vegetables and oily fish.

❖ Large reductions in tobacco smoking particularly among young people, women and people in disadvantaged communities.

❖ People keeping more physically active — by walking briskly or cycling, for example — on a regular basis.

❖ People controlling their body weight so as to keep to the right level for their physique.

❖ Avoiding drinking alcohol to excess.

The British Nutrition Foundation (2001) recommends the following:

1. Maintain a healthy body weight (BMI 20–25 kg/m^2).
2. Keep physically active.
3. Eat a healthy, balanced diet:

  • eat less fat and fatty foods
  • use vegetable oil that is high in unsaturated fat in cooking, but only in small amounts, eg. olive oil or rape-seed oil
  • eat more fruits and vegetables, at least five portions a day
  • eat more starchy foods like potatoes, rice, pasta, bread and breakfast cereals
  • choose high fibre wholemeal products
  • eat fish at least twice a week, of which one portion should be oily fish
  • choose lean meat, poultry, bread and alternatives instead of fatty meat or meat products
  • choose low-fat dairy foods, like skimmed and semi-skimmed milk or low-fat yoghurt
  • choose low-salt products and use less salt in cooking
  • drink moderately. The recommendations are three to four units per day for men and two to three units per day for women.

Wise (2001) reports a study in which it was found that a small increase in vitamin C intake could produce a substantial reduction in cardiovascular disease mortality. As stated above, physical exercise is important in reducing the risk of developing cardiovascular disease. Gottlieb (2000) reports two studies, which demonstrated that an energy expenditure of only 1000 kcals a week reduced the risk of cardiovascular disease by a 1/5th compared with those who were inactive. Furthermore, they found that it did not matter if the kcals were expended in a few long sessions or more frequent but shorter sessions. The other study which Gottlieb reports found that those who expended over 1000 kcal per week in physical activity reduced their risk by about 20% while those who expended between 500 and 999 kcals a week reduced their risk by 10%. Ludwig *et al* (1999) assert that in their ten-year longitudinal study of 2,909 healthy black and white Americans aged between eighteen and thirty, high fibre diets may protect against obesity and cardiovascular disease by lowering insulin levels. Secretion of insulin is lowered because fibre slows the rate of nutritional absorption after a meal.

Lung cancer

It is accepted that smoking is the most significant cause of lung cancer (Payne, 2001a). Lung cancer death rates lag smoking prevalence by about twenty years (Ashraf, 2002). Cigarette smoking is attributed to 80% of male and 40% of female lung cancers in the western world. In the UK, nine out of ten deaths from lung cancer in men and three in four deaths among women are estimated to be caused by smoking, accounting for 84% of all lung cancer deaths (Health Development Agency, 2001).

Lung cancer is the primary cause of premature mortality (Kanvil and Umeh, 2000) and female smokers over the age of sixty appear to have a greater risk of developing lung cancer than their counterparts (Anon, 1999). Chronic obstructive airways disease is rapidly becoming a female disease, as its prevalence is higher in women than in men. This reflects the increasing number of women now smoking compared to men.

Petty (1999) suggests that there is also a physiological reason why women smokers are more at risk of lung disease than their male counterparts:

> *Compared with men of equal size, women have smaller lungs and smaller airways. Thus, airway narrowing in response to inflammation may be more pronounced in women than in men. Women also have lower elastic recoil at any given lung volume, which compounds this effect. It is because the two factors that determine expiratory airflow, airway calibre and elastic recoil, are lower in women than in men, that women are more vulnerable to*

harmful effects of tobacco smoking on both airways and alveoli. Studies suggest that women develop chronic obstructive airways disease at lower levels of smoking than men do... Adolescents who begin smoking between ten and eighteen have impaired lung growth. Moreover, their lungs and airways never achieve normal size.

Lung cancer is said to be one of the most avoidable causes of death. Payne (2001b) reports that the World Health Organization estimates that world-wide mortality from tobacco-related diseases will rise to 10 million a year by 2030. Currently, more men than women die from lung cancer but in recent years there has been an expansion in the incidence of lung cancer and mortality in young women compared to a levelling off or decrease in the incidence in men. In developed countries there is a definite trend for increased incidence of lung cancer in women and a decrease in men. In the UK, the mortality rate for lung cancer in men has fallen since the mid-1980s, however, female rates increased until the mid-1990s at which time it seemed to level off (Payne, 2001a).

Lung cancer is the biggest killer in the UK and in the year 2000 cost the NHS about £2.5 billion. Lung cancer accounts for 25% of all lung diseases and in women has overtaken breast cancer as the leading cancer killer. It is estimated that 93% of people who are diagnosed with lung cancer are dead within five years (Mayes, 2002). Mayes asserts that women who smoke cigarettes are not only increasing their risk of developing lung cancer they may also be increasing their risk of bladder cancer.

There is a clear association between smoking, lung disease and areas of deprivation. Men and women in lower income groups and lower occupational classes have a higher incidence.

For example, the incidence rates of lung cancer among people living in the most deprived areas of Scotland are three times higher than the rates for individuals living in less deprived areas (Scottish Executive, 2001). In England and Wales, there is a higher rate of mortality from lung cancer in men in lower social economic and social groups (Payne, 2001a).

Stroke

Smoking is also associated with stroke. Hart *et al* (1999) indicate that smoking cessation results in a reduction in the risk of developing a stroke. They cite death rates from stroke in Scotland as being higher than the rest of the UK. Some 11% of male and 15% of female death rates in Scotland are due to strokes. The Stroke Association states that around 100,000 people in England and Wales have a first stroke each year, that is one every five minutes. It is estimated that around a third of people who have had a stroke will die within the first year, another third will make a good recovery and the final third will be left with moderate to severe disabilities.

The cessation of smoking seems to have a positive effect on the risk of experiencing a stroke as Hart *et al* (1999) found that former smokers had stroke rates similar to those who had never smoked. The target set by *Health in Scotland* (Scottish Executive, 2001) was to reduce smoking on Scottish adults to 31% by 2010. Siqueira *et al* (2001) report a disturbing finding that only a third of smokers have been asked by their GP to stop smoking. They continue to report that of those who had been advised to either quit or reduce their consumption, between 10% and 25% achieved the agreed goal.

Premature ageing

The smoking taskforce SCAPE claims that cigarettes can cause premature ageing and give the example of a thirty-nine-year-old woman, who has smoked for the last twenty years, having the skin of a forty-seven-year-old (Boback, 2001). The physiological reason for this is that smoking restricts blood vessels thereby reducing blood flow. A reduction in blood flow to the skin depletes the skin of oxygen and essential nutrients. It is reported that smoking may increase the production of an enzyme that breaks down collagen in the skin, which causes premature wrinkles (ASH, 2001b). The reduction in blood flow to the skin also inhibits wound healing.

Smoking in pregnancy

In the UK in 1996, one in three pregnant women smoked. Smoking in young pregnant women, particularly those from lower income groups, is particularly high. It is estimated that ten minutes of pre-natal counselling can achieve a 15% reduction in smoking rates (NHS CRD, 1999).

Toma (2001) describes the effects of smoking in utero on the foetus. Foetuses that are exposed in utero to maternal smoking are at an increased risk of asthma and being associated with a life-time of wheezing. Toma (2001) explains that this is due to physiological reasons as the foetal lung structures may be affected as they develop within the uterus leading to poor lung function after birth. There is also the possibility that there is insufficient maturation of the pulmonary immune system. Only one in four smokers succeed in stopping smoking at some point in their pregnancy.

Adverse effects occur in the second and third trimester so stopping smoking in the first trimester means the risks are the same as those for a non-smoker. According to ASH (fact sheet 7) almost 65% of women who succeed in stopping smoking while pregnant start again after the birth of the baby. The government target set in 1998 was to reduce the percentage of pregnant women smoking from 23% to 15% by 2010.

Other health-related problems associated with smoking

The Action on Smoking and Health group (ASH) illuminate a number of health-related problems attributed to smoking in their fact sheet number 7 (*Table 2.3*). Parental smoking is estimated to be responsible for at least 17,000 children, under five years of age, being admitted to hospital every year in England and Wales (NHS CRD, 1999).

Smoking cessation

> *Habit is habit and not to be flung out of the window by any man, but to be coaxed down the stairs, one step at a time.*

(Mark Twain)

Cessation of smoking is associated with a decreased risk of exacerbation of pre-existing diseases such as coronary heart disease, cancer and premature death (Froelicher and Kozuki, 2002). There are considerable health gains to be achieved from stopping smoking. Regular smokers often show high levels of motivation to quit or reduce consumption but find it very difficult to achieve this. Giving up smoking reduces the risk of myocardial infarction and some research has demonstrated that within five years of stopping smoking, the risk of a myocardial infarction is reduced to almost that of a non-smoker. By giving up smoking after a myocardial infarction the chance of recurrence can be halved. The risk of stroke decreases significantly within two years of giving up smoking and is about the same for non-smokers after five years (ASH, 2001b).

Table 2.4 for ASH (2001b) illustrates the beneficial changes, which occur when an individual stops smoking.

Table 2.3: Health-related problems associated with smoking

Health problem	Comment
Infertility	⌘ Smokers are up to three times more likely to take more than a year to conceive compared with non-smokers
Cardiovascular problems	⌘ Women who smoke and take the oral contraceptive pill have ten times the risk of developing coronary heart disease and/or cardiovascular problems
	⌘ Smoking is the cause of 90% of individuals with peripheral vascular disease having an amputation of one or both legs
Affects foetal growth and birth-weight	⌘ Babies born to mothers who smoke are on average 200 grams lighter. The more cigarettes smoked, the lower the birth weight is likely to be. Lower birth weight is associated with increased risk of death or diseases in infancy and early childhood
Perinatal mortality	⌘ Perinatal mortality, the death of a baby within the first week of life or a still birth, is increased by a third in women who smoke in pregnancy
Reduced quality and volume of breast milk	⌘ Lactating mothers who smoke have been shown to have a reduction in the fat concentration in their breast milk and the volume is likely to be less
Cervical cancer	⌘ Smokers have a four times higher risk of developing cervical cancer
Earlier onset of menopause	⌘ The natural response occurs up to two years earlier in smokers

Table 2.4: Benefits that occur from stopping smoking

Time since quitting	Beneficial health changes that take place
20 minutes	Blood pressure and pulse rate return to normal
8 hours	Nicotine and carbon monoxide levels in blood reduce by half, oxygen levels return to normal
24 hours	Carbon monoxide will be eliminated from the body Lungs start to clear out mucous and other smoking debris
48 hours	There is no nicotine left in the body Ability to taste and smell is greatly improved
72 hours	Breathing becomes easier Bronchial tubes begin to relax and energy levels increase
2–12 weeks	Circulation improves
3–9 months	Coughs, wheezing and breathing problems improve as lung function is increased by up to 10%
1 year	Risk of heart attack falls to about half that of a smoker
10 years	Risk of lung cancer falls to half that of a smoker

Why do smokers find it difficult to stop smoking?

Stopping smoking is extremely difficult and for some can be impossible (Kanvil and Umeh, 2000; Xu, 2002). It has been claimed that nicotine is more difficult to give up than heroin or cocaine (Rugkasa *et al*, 2001). Nicotine causes physiological dependency (Froelicher and Kozuki, 2002) and it has been proven beyond doubt that it is addictive (Rugkasa *et al*, 2001).

Rugkasa *et al* (2001) state that addiction is associated with stress and depression, which is accountable for almost all causes of adult smoking. They warn that by emphasising the addictive nature of tobacco it may lead to a self-fulfilling prophecy.

Addiction can be measured by how long after waking a person smokes their first cigarette of the day. In 2000, 31% of smokers had their first cigarette within fifteen minutes of waking (ASH, 2001b). Nicotine stimulates the brain to release dopamine, which is associated with pleasurable feelings. Eventually, smokers need increasing levels of nicotine to feel 'normal'. As the nicotine content of their blood drops below a certain level, they begin to crave for a cigarette. This craving makes the smoker feel 'stressed' until the craving is relieved. The relief when this craving is finally satisfied is the feeling that smokers commonly mistake as 'relaxing' (ASH, 2001b).

Rugkasa *et al*'s 2001 qualitative study aim was to explore the understanding that ten- and eleven-year-olds have of tobacco addiction at an age where experimenting with cigarettes often starts. They conducted eighty-five focus interviews with forty-one males and forty-four females in economically deprived areas of Northern Ireland. Three participants reported smoking regularly, twenty had already smoked experimentally and one participant stated that they were addicted. The results of the study suggest that the notion of tobacco consumption is something that symbolically belongs to the world of adults. They believed that addiction only happened in adults and the majority of children knew it was wrong to smoke and most held negative views about children who did smoke. When asked by Rugkasa *et al* (2001) what the negative consequences of smoking were, the children stated the following: yellow fingers; black lungs; cancer; reduced fitness; waste of money and risk of being caught by parents. The latter was viewed as the most dramatic consequence. Rugkasa *et al* found that the reason why children started smoking was related to direct peer pressure and the fact that children smoke to improve their status among friends and peers to maintain social relations. This reflects findings from Koivusilta *et al* (1999) who state that sharing a habit like smoking adds to social cohesion and the habit becoming a source of self-esteem and self-image. Froelicher and Kozuki (2002) conclude that research findings consistently reveal that high perceived self-efficacy predicts the individual's success in quitting or maintaining smoking cessation. According to Bandura (1997) self-efficacy are people's judgements of their capabilities to carry something out.

Hunt *et al* (2000) discovered in their study that people who believe that they have a family history of heart disease and see themselves at risk of the disease are far less likely to smoke. They conclude that understanding a person's construction of familial risk of heart disease is important for health promotion and that it is linked to behavioural risk factors.

Strategies to help cessation of smoking

The motivation to stop smoking is often related to a perceived threat to an individual's health and the perception that stopping smoking will eliminate that threat (Kanvil and Umeh, 2000). It is known that stopping smoking post myocardial infarction is associated with a significant decrease in mortality and markedly reduces the readmission rates related to coronary heart disease (Hajek *et al*, 2002).

Since a perceived threat can be a strong motivating factor it is concerning that a survey conducted by Dawe and Goddard in 1997 revealed that only 38% of current smokers could recall ever being given advice to stop smoking by their GP (NHS CRD, 1999). An important aspect to consider in promoting smoking cessation is an understanding of the reasons behind commencing smoking and the socio-cultural milieu in which it takes place.

Smoking behaviour is a complex issue, which involves behavioural, social, cultural and economic factors (Froelicher and Kozuki, 2002). Socially and economically deprived groups are more likely to smoke (Graham and Der, 1999; Wiltshire *et al*, 2001). The cessation rates for the better off almost doubled during 1970–1990, whereas the cessation rates in the poorer groups have remained relatively consistent over the same timespan (Graham and Der, 1999). Koivusilta *et al* (1999) and Pavis and Cunningham-Burley (1999) note that there is an association between higher rates of smoking and such factors as low self-esteem, low academic ability, poor social support, inadequate family bonding and/or functioning. In families where the parents or siblings smoke there is a higher rate of taking up smoking in children. Furthermore, if the child's best friend smokes or there is a belief that the smoking rate is high in their peer group, there is a high association that the child will start smoking (Pavis and Cunningham-Burley, 1999).

Pavis and Cunningham-Burley (1999) conducted a two-year ethnographic study involving 106 young people. Data were collected through participant observation and semi-structured interviews. They found that asking for a cigarette was repeatedly used as a way of encouraging a longer conversation and this behaviour was markedly obvious when the individual wanted to join a larger group or when members of the opposite sex approached one another. Moreover, they found that in street smoking, cigarettes were nearly always shared and Pavis and Cunningham-Burley (1999) assert that this served to strengthen social bonds.

There is also an association with smoking and stress. Bastian *et al* (2001) suggest that high job demands and stressful working environments may trigger persistent smoking. They note that the association is higher with job strain as opposed to home strain and that women who smoke are likely to be single, have less educational qualifications and report higher levels of job strain. They suggest that the social support gained by living with a partner may be the reason why these women are less likely to smoke. It is reported by Kanvil and Umeh (2000) that women use cigarettes as a buffer against negative feelings, whereas men tend to smoke out of habit or to bolster positive feelings.

One of the Government's priorities is a reduction in smoking among low-income groups and it is also a key element of its strategy for tackling health inequalities (Scottish Executive, 1999; DoH, 1998; DoH, 1999). Obviously there are a number of strategies which can be used in helping people to stop smoking, and these are now discussed.

Legislation

Watson (2001) reported on the negotiations between members of Scottish Parliament (MSPs) and the European Union in respects to changes in legislation on smoking. Watson reports that the MSPs wanted tougher health warnings on cigarette packets. For example, they wanted a ban on the use of the terms low tar, light and mild; the size of warning labels increased to 40% on the front and 50% on the back and new messages being used such as:

> *Passive smoking harms those around you, especially children.*
>
> *Smoking kills half a million people each year in the European Union.*
>
> *Smoking causes cancer and heart disease.*

The draft legislation suggested by the members of the European Parliament (MEPs) would also reduce the maximum tar content per cigarette from 12mgs to 10mgs, nicotine levels to 1mg and for the first time, the introduction of a 10mg limit for carbon monoxide. As Watson (2001) reports, the MEPs draft legislation went further than the EU ministers wanted but they were prepared to support about a third of the recommendations. As yet, which recommendation will be supported is unknown.

Norway, Finland and Iceland all introduced advertising bans in the 1970s which had the effect of reducing smoking rates. Norway has significantly lower smoking rates than the UK (Ashraf, 2002). In Eire, they have introduced tougher tobacco laws. They have banned the selling of cigarettes in packets of tens; banned sponsorship by the tobacco industry and they want to increase the age at which tobacco products can be sold from sixteen to eighteen years of age. They have also introduced free nicotine replacement therapy to individuals who are means tested medical cardholders (Payne, 2001b).

Banning smoking in public places

The effects of restricting smoking in public places is associated with a reduction in the daily smoking rate and an increase in cessation rates (Wakefield *et al*, 2000). Wakefield *et al* (2000) argue that as smoking restrictions become more pervasive, smoking will be perceived as more socially unacceptable and inconvenient. They also assert that by banning smoking at home, even if adults smoke, it sets a good example to children and reduces the likelihood of their taking up smoking. Jarvis *et al* (2001) believe that this would also reduce passive smoking.

Restricting smoking in public sector and workplaces causes smokers to go outside to smoke. Individuals smoking outside are more likely to smoke faster with more frequent and deeper inhalations regardless of nicotine dependency (Payne, 2001b). Docherty *et al* (1999) note that large workplaces are more likely than smaller ones to restrict smoking, but they are also more likely to provide cessation support for their employees. There is evidence that the general population is becoming increasingly in favour of restricting smoking in public places. A survey by the Office for National Statistics (2001) found that more than 80% of people polled in the UK would support restricting smoking in places of work, restaurants, banks and post-offices. More than 50% would be in favour of a smoking ban in public houses. This is positive since it is reported that passive smoking is associated with an increased risk of stroke in men and women. Just thirty minutes can affect the blood flow through the heart (ASH, 2001b). Passive smoking in children causes an increased risk in a number of illnesses such as respiratory tract infections, asthma, middle ear infection, cardiovascular impairment and behavioural problems (ASH, 2001b).

Role of health education in smoking cessation

There should be more health education, advice and support available as individuals attempt to cut down or give up smoking. Interventions should act directly on socio-economic and psychological environments, which serve to work against successful cessation occurring (Graham and Der, 1999).

Lawn *et al* (2002) point out that smoking cessation for people who have a concurrent mental health problem is extremely low (Lawn *et al*, 2002) and smoking relapse is more likely to occur in people in low mood states.

In their randomised controlled trial, Hajek *et al* (2002) involved 540 smokers who were post myocardial infarction or cardiac surgery with seventeen English hospitals. The participants were randomised into the control group which received the normal care of brief verbal advice and a booklet and the intervention group, which received twenty to thirty minutes of contact with others giving up smoking, a special booklet, a quiz, a carbon monoxide reading test and a declaration of commitment to give up smoking. Both groups were followed up at six weeks and again at a year and continuations of cessation of smoking were measured by self-report and blood biochemical analysis. The results indicated that at six weeks, of the control group, 59% (n=151) remained abstinent compared with 60% (n=159) of the intervention group. At a year, 41% (n=102) of the control group remained abstinent compared to 37% (n=94) of the intervention group. The researchers concluded that a single session delivered along with routine care had insufficient power to influence highly dependent smokers. They therefore advocated that smoking cessation involved more intensive training and rehearsal.

West (2002) reports a Cochrane review which clearly demonstrated that behavioural support and counselling improves the smoker's chance of achieving lasting abstinence. This type of treatment must be provided by specifically trained personnel who are employed for this purpose and are not expected to fulfil this role as well as fitting it into other jobs (West, 2002).

Bovet *et al* (2002) conducted a randomised controlled trial in which 153 smokers participated. All participants received smoking cessation counselling. The experimental group (n=74) received ultra-soundography of their carotid and femoral arteries. Following this procedure, they were provided with a photograph of the ultrasonic image demonstrating their own atherosclerotic lesions and an explanation of what this meant for them as an individual. Their findings demonstrated a quit rate of 22% in the experimental group, compared to 6% in the control group. The value of personalised information and materials as being more effective than standardised materials was noted by Lancaster *et al* in 2000.

In terms of promoting change in behaviour, Prochaska and DiClemente's (1983) five stages of change cited by Froelicher and Kozuki (2002) offers a useful approach. Froelicher and Kozuki (2002) take each stage and suggest corresponding actions.

Stage	Prochaska and DiClemente (1983)	Froelicher and Kozuki (2002)
1	Pre-contemplation	Help person to think seriously about quitting over the next six months
2	Contemplation	Tip the balance so that the cons outweigh the pros
3	Action	Help person to plan a quit attempt
4	Maintenance	Support person in taking steps to change
5	Relapse	Identify and use relapse prevention strategies

Those people whose work involves health and health promotion are ideally placed to influence many smokers (Gorin, 2001). Gorin

(2001) reports that the majority of nurses believe that they have a responsibility to counsel patients regarding their smoking but only 50% of hospitalised patients report that they have received advice to stop smoking from a nurse or, indeed, a health professional. Gorin (2001) suggests that this may be due to a lack of confidence in the health professional's skill to provide preventative care. Gorin (2001) conducted a cross-sectional survey of 476 junior and senior student nurses in twelve schools of nursing in the New York area. The aim of the survey was to determine nurses' knowledge of tobacco control, beliefs and practices. She found that 76% of students report that they practice tobacco control. There was an interesting difference between students who smoked and those who did not. Current smokers were less likely to practice tobacco control with patients while those who did not smoke had better knowledge of smoking cessation approaches and were more confident in their smoking cessation skills. Students who smoked were less likely to perceive themselves to be role models or health educators.

Gorin's (2001) findings are not isolated to nurses. Wyn and Solis (2001) report that doctor-patient discussion of smoking cessation were inconsistent. They report that 60% of female patients did not receive information about stopping smoking when attending their GP. It is reported that advice from health professionals about quitting can achieve cessation rates of up to 2%; however, if the advice is accompanied by the use of nicotine replacement therapy (NRT), then the quit rate rises to 12%.

The time taken to give the advice is estimated to be three minutes and considering that a large number of smokers are in contact with health professionals, incorporating this advice into their daily practice would lead to a substantial health gain (NHS CRD 1999). Anderson *et al* (2002) asserts that a three- to ten-minute counselling session by a physician is likely to produce a response of approximately 16% of patients quitting.

Wiltshire *et al* (2001) conducted a cross-sectional qualitative study in two deprived areas in Edinburgh, Scotland. They randomly selected from GP lists fifty females and fifty males between the ages of twenty-five and forty. Data were collected using semi-structured interviews. Wiltshire *et al* found that most of those they interviewed wished to stop smoking, but the importance of smoking in their daily lives and their addiction to nicotine were major barriers. They assert that those in deprived areas view the ready availability of cheap, smuggled cigarettes as a means of dealing with increasing costs of cigarettes. Wiltshire suggest that up to 25%–30% of cigarettes consumed in the UK are contraband and that this only serves to undermine cessation services which specifically target low income smokers. It is estimated that one in every three cigarettes smoked in the UK are smuggled, which accounts for £3.8 billion lost in taxes (HDA, undated).

Woods and Mitchell (1997) state that in exploring reasons why women do not use smoking cessation programmes, the following barriers were identified:

- managing their lives in highly stressful environments
- experiencing major isolation within their environments
- smoking viewed as pleasurable and attainable within limited financial resources
- perceived minimal health risk related to smoking
- commonality of smoking with their communities
- scarcity of information about the process of cessation
- belief that all that was needed was self-determination.

The HDA (undated) reports that individuals from the lower socio-economic groups have less successful cessation rates than those in higher socio-economic groups. The difference is not due to motivation, but the level of addiction to nicotine. Poorer smokers tend both to choose to smoke more and to smoke each cigarette more intensively, thereby achieving higher levels of nicotine in their blood stream.

Smoking cessation clinics

In their White Paper, *Smoking Kills* (1998), the Government set out policies for addressing smoking as one of the major causes of stroke and coronary heart disease. They set up a three-year public education campaign costing up to £50 million, banned advertising of tobacco advertising and set aside £60 million, again over three years, for smoking cessation services in deprived areas known as health action zones (HAZs). Health action zones are designed to facilitate a synergy between all those contributing to the health of the local population to design and implement strategies (Jacobson and Yen, 1998). Smoking cessation clinics were launched in health action zones in 1999/2000. These services were rolled out across the NHS in 2000/2001. In the three years up to and including 2001/2002, £53 million has been made available for these services and a further £20 million is available for 2002/2003 (DoH, 2002).

What happens at smoking cessation clinics? Individuals receive one-to-one support from a trained adviser and can attend local support groups. With their adviser, individuals set a quit date, learn how to cope with cravings and pick up health tips. They will normally be offered a choice of smoking cessation aids, such as nicotine replacement therapy or Zyban with the view to reducing cravings and withdrawal symptoms as this has been shown to increase the chances of cessation. Nicotine replacement therapy (NRT) is available in a number of forms: transdermal patches, chewing gum, nasal spray and inhalers. It works by releasing a steady dose of nicotine into the bloodstream, easing the withdrawal symptoms. Zyban is a drug that suppresses the part of the brain that provides smokers with their 'nicotine buzz'. It also reduces cravings and withdrawal symptoms (DoH, 2002b).

Nicotine replacement therapy is constantly found to be effective, however, there persists a concern over its use in individuals with coronary heart disease. Froelicher and Kozuki (2002) report studies and expert opinion, which advise that the risks of smoking in cardiac patients far outweigh the risks of using nicotine replacement therapy. QUIT, the UK Charity that helps people give up smoking, states that nicotine replacement therapy products can improve a person's chances of stopping smoking by up to four times. They provide a very useful service and offer practical advice on ways to stop smoking. Nicotine replacement therapy is now available on prescription and normally reinforced by smoking cessation support services (Scottish Executive, 2001).

The DoH (2002a) produced the following statistics on smoking cessation in England between April and September 2001. 104,800 people set a date to quit smoking through smoking cessation services. Following a four-week follow-up, 53,500 had successfully quit, representing 51% of those who had set a quit date.

The DoH (2000b) sets a target of reducing smoking rates among manual groups from 32% in 1998 to 26% by 2010. The HDA (2001) argue that smoking cessation services are highly effective and particularly effective in reaching low-income smokers. Smoking cessation services (ASH, 2001b) advocate fifteen tips for stopping smoking (see overleaf). Details related to the tips can be found on http://www.ash.org.uk/html/factsheets/html/fact24.html.

Froelicher and Kozuki (2002) advocate identification of cognitive and behavioural strategies to cope with situations. For example, if they are in the habit of smoking after a meal, then adopt one of the following strategies: move away from the table; take a small walk; brush teeth. The emphasis is on relapse prevention through rehearsing coping responses and strategies (Froelicher and Kozuki, 2002).

Tips for stopping smoking

1. Get professional help.
2. Prepare mentally.
3. Demolish smoking myths.
4. Understand what to expect.
5. Make a list of reasons why you want to stop smoking.
6. Consider the money.
7. Set a date.
8. Involve friends or family.
9. Deal with nicotine withdrawal.
10. Other treatments may help.
11. Find a (temporary) substitute habit.
12. Deal with any weight gain worries.
13. Avoid temptation.
14. Stop completely.
15. Watch out for relapse.

Smoking low tar/nicotine cigarettes does not eliminate health risks (Froelicher and Kozuki, 2002). Indeed, Payne (2001c) suggests that switching from high to low tar causes people to compensate for the reduced levels of nicotine by increasing the number of puffs and the depth of inhalation. This changes the part of lungs most affected by smoking and corresponding with an increasing rate of adeno-carcinoma development.

Smoking cessation message for adolescents

It is now considered most important to target health promotion strategies at children and adolescents before cigarette use is firmly established, as opposed to older groups whose addiction makes cessation more difficult (Kanvil and Umeh, 2000). According to ASH (2001b) only 1% of eleven-year-olds are regular smokers but this rises to 23% of fifteen-year-olds. Eighty-two per cent of smokers take up the habit as teenagers. The NHS CRD (1999) recommended that children between four and eight should be targeted rather than eleven- to seventeen-year-olds because by the time a child has reached the age of eleven their attitudes and experimentation with smoking has already occurred. The White Paper, *Smoking Kills*, identified young people as a priority and set targets to reduce smoking in this group in England from 13% to 9% or less by 2010. Paavola *et al* (2001) report that several studies have identified that young people have a desire to quit and that many attempt to do so but are often unsuccessful. They continue by asserting that whether the cessation attempt is successful or not is strongly dependent on how much their peers smoke.

The stimulus for smoking cessation in young people is usually associated with their health or financial reasons. There are also indications that significant others, such as girlfriends or boyfriends, can provide a stimulus to quit (Paavola *et al*, 2001). In their study, Paavola *et al* (2001) discovered that smoking cessation was more common if the best friend was a non-smoker; in individuals who were married and employed; in individuals who consumed less alcohol and those who had engaged in leisure activities.

The NHS CRD (1999) identified four prevention strategies for use in young people. These are:

- school-based programmes
- mass media
- retailer interventions
- community interventions.

School-based programmes have moved from scare tactics to a focus on providing young people with skills to resist the pressures to smoke: a strategy that seems to be more effective than the scare tactic which was used previously.

The website: http://www.giving_upsmoking.co.uk provides some useful phrases and tactics for young people to use. For example:

Not just at the moment. When I want to shorten my life a little, I'll give you a call.

Not for me. If I want to avoid pulling sometime though, I'll let you know.

Mass media is an increasingly popular method, as television is believed to influence young people's perceptions of the real word and acceptable social behaviour. It also helps develop cultural norms. Naidoo and Wills (2001) assert that the mass media helps in a variety of ways such as promoting and legitimising and triggering activity in key issues. They cite the example of the national 'No Smoking' day which results in 1% of the population's smokers quitting smoking for three months or more.

Retailer interventions involve retailers abiding by the law and not selling cigarettes to anyone under sixteen years of age. The NHS CRD (1999) report the findings of a survey which found that 25% of secondary school children had tried to buy cigarettes at shops in the last year. Only 38% of these individuals had been refused at least once. Community interventions include age restrictions for tobacco purchase, smoke-free public places, media campaigns and special programmes in schools.

The NHS CRD (1999) conclude that a multi-faceted approach is required and the importance of the school environment needs to be recognised.

'Smokebusters' is a community-based smoking prevention initiative for young people which aims to prevent them from starting to smoke. This initiative was first introduced in 1985 and the numbers have gradually increased in the UK and Europe over the last decade. The first one was called 'Project Smoke Free' but after a competition involving the young people, a ten-year-old suggested 'Smokebusters' as a name. The philosophy of the club is to promote not smoking as being a desirable adult choice. Membership of the club means that young people have a strong supportive peer group which helps to provide information and support in rejecting smoking in ways so as not to lose face. Teijlingen and Bruce (1999) report that there is a significant rise in children's knowledge and more negative attitudes towards smoking. There is, as yet, no direct evidence that being a member of such clubs affects a behavioural change although it is known that there is a delay in the onset of smoking.

It is good to emphasise that young people can avoid nicotine addiction by not smoking. According to Meyrick (2001), this is a powerful message as it focuses on the loss of autonomy that comes with taking up smoking: focusing on the threat of addiction is more likely to have greater immediacy to adolescents than focusing on longer-term health risks caused by smoking (Meyrick, 2001). Meyrick (2001) warns that the tone and framing of messages to adolescents must be positive and strongly advocates focusing on the benefits of not smoking as opposed to the vivid consequences of smoking.

Suggested web resources

http://www.ash.org.uk
http://www.bbc.co.uk/health/kth/stop.shtml BBC Health: Kick the Habit
http://www.givingupsmoking.co.uk
http://www.cdc.gov/tobacco US CDC tobacco information and prevention source
http://www.cdc.gov/tobacco.sgr/sgr4kids/sgrmenu.htm US Surgeon General's Report about
    Kids and Smoking
http://www.idrc.ca/tobacco/en/index.html Research for International Tobacco Control
http://www.quitnet.com QuitNet
http://www.quitnow.info.au — not for the faint hearted — gory pictures of what smoking
    does to various organs
http://tobacco.who.int WHO Tobacco-Free Initiative

References

Amos A, Haglund M (2000) From social taboo to 'torch of freedom': the marketing of
    cigarettes to women. *Tobacco Control* 9: 3–8

Anderson JE, Jorenby DE, Scott WJ, Fiore MC (2002) Treating tobacco use and
    dependence: an evidence-based clinical practice guideline for tobacco cessation. *Chest*
    121(3): 686–7

Anon (1999) Lung cancer risk greater in women. *Women's Health in Primary Care* 2(12):
    919

Action on Smoking and Health (2001a) *Smoking and Health Inequalities*. ASH, NHS Health
    Development Agency, London

Action on Smoking and Health (2001b) Fact Sheets. ASH, NHS Health Development
    Agency, London

Ashraf H (2002) European tobacco control reaches a critical phase. *Lancet* 359: 585–6

Bandura A (1997) The anatomy of change. (editorial). *Am J Health Promotion* 12(1): 8–10

Barnard RJ, Inkeles SB (1999) Effects of an intensive diet and exercise program on lipids in
    postmenopausal women. *Women's Health* 9(3): 155–61

Barrett S (2001) Improving access and quality for ethnic minority women. *Women's Health*
    11(4): 345–54

Bastian LA, Owens SS, Kim H, Barnett LR, Seigler IC (2001) Cigarette Smoking in Veteran
    Women: The Impact of Job Strain. *Women's Health Issues* 11(2): 103–9

Boback A (2001) *Smoking can add years*. http://www.health-secure.net (accessed March
    2002)

Bovet P, Perret F, Cornuz J, Quilindo J, Paccaud F (2002) Improved smoking cessation in
    smokers given ultrasound photographs of their own atherosclerotic plaques.
    Preventative Medicine 34: 215–20

Brink E, Karlson BW, Hallberg LRM (2002) Health experiences of first-time myocardial
    infarction: factors influencing women's and men's health-related quality of life after
    five months. *Psychology, Health and Medicine* 7(1): 5–16

British Heart Foundation (2002) *Coronary Heart Disease Statistics*.
    http://www.dphpc.ox.uk/bhfthprg/stats/2000/2002/keyfacts/index.html (accessed
    February 2002)

British Nutrition Foundation (BNF) (2001) *Coronary Heart Disease.* http://www.nutrition.org.uk (accessed March 2002)

Cancer Working Group (1999) *Strategic Priorities in Cancer Research and Development.* http://www.doh.gov.uk/research/document/rd3/cancer_final_report.pdf (accessed March 2002)

Charlton A, Bates C (2000) Decline in teenage smoking with rise in mobile phone ownership: hypothesis. *Br Med J* **321**: 1155

Coleman JC, Hendry LB (1999) *The Nature of Adolescence.* 3rd edn. Routledge, London

Dawe F, Goddard E (1997) *Smoking-related behaviours and attitudes. A report on research using the ONS omnibus survey produced on behalf of the Department of Health.* The Stationery Office, London

Doherty G, Fraser E, Hardin J (1999) Health promotion in the Scottish workplace: a case for moving the goalposts. *Health Educ Res* **14**(4): 565–73

Department of Health (1992) *The Health of the Nation: A strategy for health in England.* DoH, London

Department of Health (1998) *Smoking Kills.* Stationery Office, London

Department of Health (1999) *Saving Lives: Our Healthier Nation.* DoH, London

Department of Health (2001a) *The Annual Report of the Chief Medical Officer of the Department of Health 2001: On the State of the Public Health.* DoH, London

Department of Health (2001b) *Priorities and Planning Framework.* 2002/2003. http://www.doh.gov.uk/planning2002-2003 (accessed February 2002)

Department of Health (2002a) *Statistics on smoking cessation services in Health Authorities: England, April to September 2001.* http://www.doh.gov.uk/public/smokingapril01.html (accessed February 2002)

Department of Health (2002b) *Inside story: Smoking — give up for good.* http://www.doh.gov.uk/newsdesk/inside/mar2002/index.html (accessed February 2002)

Duvernoy CS, Eagle KA (2000) Diagnosing and treating acute myocardial infarction in women. *Women's Health in Primary Care* **4**(8): 542–56

Flay BR (1993) Youth tobacco use: Risks, patterns, and control. In: Orleans CT, Slade J, eds. *Nicotine Addiction: Principles and management.* Oxford University Press, New York: 365–84

Froelicher ES, Kozuki Y (2002) Theoretical applications of smoking cessation interventions to individuals with medical conditions: women's initiative for non-smoking (WINS) — Part III. *Int J Nurs Stud* **39**: 1–15

Gabhainn SN, Kelleher CC, Naughton AM, Carter F, Flanagan M, McGrath MJ (1999) Socio-demographic variations in perspectives on cardiovascular disease and associated risk factors. *Health Educ Res* **14**(5): 619–28

Garber CE (1997) The benefits of physical activity on coronary heart disease and coronary heart disease risk factors in women. *Women's Health Issues* **7**(1): 17–23

Gorin SS (2001) Predictors of tobacco control among nursing students. *Patient Education and Counselling* **44**: 251–62

Gottlieb S (2000) Short, sharp bouts of exercise good for the heart. *Br Med J* **321**: 589

Graham H, Der G (1999) Patterns and predictors of tobacco consumption among women. *Health Educ Ress* **14**(5): 611–18

Hajek P, Taylor TZ, Mills P (2002) Brief intervention during hospital admission to help patients to give up smoking after myocardial infarction and bypass surgery: randomised controlled trial. *Br Med J* **324**: 1–6

Hart CL, Hole DJ, Smith GD (1999) Risk factors and 20-year stroke mortality in men and women in the Renfrew/Paisley study in Scotland. *Stroke* **30**: 1999–2007

Health Development Agency (2001) Research and Evidence. http://www.hda-online.org.uk/html/research/effectivenessreviews/html (accessed February 2002)

Health Development Agency (2001) *Coronary Heart Disease: Guidance for implementing the preventive aspects of the National Service Framework*. http://www.hda-online.org.uk/documents/chdframework.pdf (accessed February 2002)

Hine D (2001) National perspective: United Kingdom. *Women's Health* 11(4): 293–9

Holliday JE, Lowe JM, Outram S (2000) Women's experience of myocardial infarction. *Int J Nurs Practice* 6: 307–16

Hunt K, Davison C, Emslie C, Ford G (2000) Are perceptions of a family history of heart disease related to health-related attitudes and behaviour? *Health Educ Res* 15(2): 131–43

Jacobson B, Yen L (1998) Health action zones. *Br Med J* 316:164

Jarvis MJ, Feyerabend C, Bryant A, Hedges B, Primatesta P (2001) Passive smoking in the home: plasma cotine concentrations in non-smokers with smoking partners. *Tobacco Control* 10: 368–74

Josefson D (2001) Study links passive smoking and coronary blood flow. *Br Med J* 323: 252

Kanvil N, Umeh KF (2000) Lung cancer and cigarette use: Cognitive factors, protection motivation and past behaviour. *Br J Health Psychol* 5: 235–48

Koivusilta LK, Rimpela AH, Rimpela MK (1999) Health-related lifestyle in adolescence — origin of social class differences in health? *Health Educ Res* 14(3): 339–55

Lancaster T, Stead L, Silagy C, Sowden A (2000) Effectiveness of interventions to help people stop smoking: findings from the Cochrane Library. *Br Med J* 321: 355–8

Lawn SJ, Pols RG, Barber JG (2002) Smoking and quitting: a qualitative study with community-living psychiatric clients. *Soc Sci Med* 54(1): 93–104

Lee C (1998) *Women's Health: Psychological and Social Perspectives*. Sage, London

Ludwig DS *et al* (1999) Dietary fibre, weight gain and cardiovascular disease risk factors in young adults. *J Am Med Assoc* 282: 1539–46

MacIntyre K, Stewart S, Chalmers J, Pell A, Finlayson A, Boyd J, Redpath A, McMurray J, Capewell S (2001) Relation between socioeconomic deprivation and death from a first myocardial infarction in Scotland: population based analysis. *Br Med J* 322: 1152–3

Mayes R (2002) *Easing the burden of lung disease*. http://www.health-news.co.uk (accessed February 2002)

McCool JP, Cameron LD, Petrie KJ (2001) Adolescent perceptions of smoking imagery in film. *Soc Sci Med* 52:1557–87

Meyrick J de (2001) Forget the 'blood and gore': an alternative message strategy to help adolescents avoid cigarette smoking. *Health Educ* 101(3): 99–107

Mind Out for Mental Health. http://www.mindout.net (accessed February 2002)

Moffat BM, Johnson JL (2001) Through the haze of cigarettes: Teenage girls' stories about cigarette addiction. *Qualitative Health Res* 11(5): 668–81

Moher M, Yudkin P, Wright LW, Turner R, Fuller A, Schofield T *et al* (2001) Children's emotional and behavioural well-being and family environment: findings from the Health Survey for England. *Soc Sci Med* 53: 423–440

Naidoo J, Wills J (2001) *Health Studies: An Introduction*. Palgrave, Hampshire

National Health Service Centre for Reviews and Dissemination (1999) Preventing the uptake of smoking in young people. *Effective Health Care* 5(5): 1–12

National Health Service R & D Strategic Review (1999) Cornonary Heart Disease and Stroke: Report of Topic Working Group. http://www.doh.gov.uk/research/documents/rd3/cvds_final_report.pdf (accessed February 2002)

Office for National Statistics (2001) http://www.health-secure.net (accessed February 2002)

Oxley GM (2001) HIV/AIDS knowledge and self-esteem among adolescents. *Clin Nurs Res* **10**(2): 214–24

Paavola M, Vartiainen E, Puska P (2001) Smoking cessation between teenage years and adulthood. *Health Educ Res* **16**(1): 49–57

Pavis S, Cunningham-Burley S (1999) Male youth street culture: understanding the context of health related behaviours. *Health Educ Res* **14**(5): 583–96

Payne D (2001a) Ireland to introduce tougher tobacco law. *Br Med J* **322**: 574

Payne S (2001b) 'Smoke like a man, die like a man'? A review of the relationship between gender, sex and lung cancer. *Soc Sci Med* **53**: 1067–80

Petty TL (1999) The rising epidemic of COAD in women. *Women's Health in Primary Care* **2**(12): 942–50

Pocock SJ, McCormack V, Gueyffier F, Boutitie F, Fagard RH, Boissel JP (2001) A score for predicting risk of death from cardiovascular disease in adults with raised blood pressure, based on individual patient data from randomised controlled trials. *Br Med J* **323**: 75–81

Prochaska JO, DiClemente DCC (1983) Stages and processes of self-change of smoking: toward an integrated model of change. *J Consult Clin Psychol* **51**(3): 390–5

Richardson K, Crosier A (undated) *Smoking and Health Inequalities*. Health Development Agency and ASH, London. http://www.hda-online.org.uk/downloads.pdfs (accessed February 2002)

Rousseau ME (2001) Evidence-based practice in women's health: hormone therapy for women at menopause. *J Midwif Women's Health* **46**(3): 167–80

Rugkasa J, Knox B, Sittlington J, Kennedy O, Treacy MP, Abaunze PS (2001) Anxious adults vs. cool children: children's views on smoking and addiction. *Soc Sci Med* **53**: 593–602

Sacks FM *et al* (2001) Effects on blood pressure of reduced dietary sodium and the dietary approaches to stop hypertension (DASH) diet. *New Engl J Med* **344**: 3–10

Sargent JD, Beach ML, Dalton MA, Mott LA, Tickle JJ, Aherns MB, Heatherton TF (2001) Effect of seeing tobacco use in films on trying smoking among adolescents: cross sectional study. *Br Med J* **323**: 1–6

Scottish Executive (2001) *Health in Scotland*. http://www.show.scot.nhs.uk/publications (accessed February 2002,)

Schifrin E (2001) An overview of women's health issues in the United States and United Kingdom. *Women's Health Issues* **11**(4): 261–81

Secretary of State for Scotland (1999) *Towards a Healthier Scotland*. HMSO, Edinburgh

Siqueira LM, Rolnitzy LM, Rickert VI (2001) Smoking cessation in adolescents: the role of nicotine dependence, stress, and coping methods. *Arch Pediatr Adolesc Med* **155**(4): 489–95

Smith GD, Chaturvedi N, Harding S, Nazroo J, Williams R (2000) Ethnic inequalities in health: a review of UK epidemiological evidence. *Crit Public Health* **10**(4): 375–408

Spear H, Kulbok PA (2001) Adolescent health behaviours and related factors: a review. *Public Health Nurs* **18**(2): 82–93

Teijlingen EV, Bruce J (1999) Systematic reviews of health promotion initiatives — the Smokebusters experience. *Health Educ* **2**: 76–83

Tod AM, Read C, Lacey A, Abott J (2001) Barriers to uptake of services for coronary heart disease: qualitative study. *Br Med J* **323**: 1–5

Toma T (2001) Exposure in utero to maternal smoking increases risk of asthma. *Br Med J* **322**: 450

van Tiel D, van Vliet KP, Moerman CJ (1998) Sex differences in illness beliefs and illness behaviour in patients with suspected coronary artery disease. *Patient Educ Counselling* **33**: 143–7

Wakefield MA, Chaloupka FJ, Kaufman NJ, Orleans T, Barker DC, Ruel, EE (2000) Effect of restrictions on smoking at home, at school, and in public places on teenage smoking: cross sectional study. *Br Med J* **321**: 333–7

Wallis EJ, Ramsay LE, Haq IU, Ghahramani P, Jackson PR, Rowland-Yeo K, Yeo WE (2000) Coronary and cardiovascular risk estimation from primary prevention: validation of a new Sheffield table in the 1995 Scottish health survey population. *Br Med J* **321**: 671–6

Watson R (2001) MEPs back tougher health warnings on cigarette packets. *Br Med J* **322**: 7

West R (2002) Helping patients in hospital quit smoking. *Br Med J* **324**: 64

Wiles R, Kinmonth A (2001) Patients' understandings of heart attack: implications for prevention of recurrence. *Patient Educ Counselling* **44**: 161–9

Wiltshire S, Bancroft A, Amos A, Parry O (2001) They're doing people a service — qualitative study of smoking, smuggling and social deprivation. *Br Med J* **323**: 203–7

Wise J (2001) Small rise in vitamin C intake could greatly reduce heart disease. *Br Med J* **323**: 576

Woods MF, Mitchell ES (1997) Preventative Health Issues: The perimenopausal to mature years (45–64). In: Allen KM, Phillips JM, eds. *Women's Health: Across the lifespan.* Lippincott, Philadelphia: chapter 5

Wyn R, Solis B (2001) Women's health issues across the lifespan. *Women's Health Issues* **11**(3): 148–59

Xu KT (2002) Compensating behaviors, regret, and heterogeneity in the dynamics of smoking behaviour. *Soc Sci Med* **54**: 133–46

3

Maintaining a healthy diet and weight

Introduction

Obesity and being overweight is an increasing problem world-wide. The prevalence rates have increased dramatically over the last two decades. The WHO has declared obesity a global epidemic (Atkinson and Nitzke, 2001). This chapter focuses on the health consequences of being overweight or obese and a variety of health promotion activities are discussed. Barriers to adopting healthy eating behaviours and suggested interventions relevant to both adults and young people are explored.

Obesity and being overweight

The report from the National Audit Office states that nearly two thirds of men and half of women in England are overweight or obese. People in lower socio-economic groups, women and black Caribbean and Pakistani women are most at risk (www.nao.gov.uk). Levels of obesity are lower in Bangladeshi and Chinese women but higher in black Caribbean and Pakistani women. All female minority ethnic groups have levels of central obesity well above that of the general female population, with black Caribbean and Pakistani women two times and Bangladeshi women over three times as likely to have central obesity compared to those in the general population (BNF, 2001).

Overweight and obesity increases with age. In the age group sixteen to twenty-four, 27% of women are overweight or obese compared with 68% in the age group fifty-five to sixty-four. Central obesity also increases with age, particularly in men. In women over fifty-five years of age the rate is about 23% compared with 7% in the sixteen to thirty-four age range. Both genders in unskilled occupations are over four times as likely as those in professional employment to be classed as morbidly obese (BMI >40) (BHF, 2002).

Particularly worrying is the increasing rate of overweight and obese children and adolescents. The prevalence rates in children are reported to range from 6% to 17%. In a study conducted by Rudolf *et al* (2001) in which 694 school pupils took part, it is reported that these children had their height, weight and skinfold thickness measurement taken for three consecutive years. Rudolf *et al* (2001) found that for girls, 22% (n=56) of nine-year-olds were overweight compared to 32% of eleven-year-olds. In terms of obesity, 10% (n=27) of the nine-year-old girls were obese compared to 13% (n=15) of the eleven-year-olds. The figures for the boys were as follows: 22% (n=71) of nine-year-old boys were considered overweight compared to 27% (n=41) of eleven-year-olds; and 10% (n=33) of nine-year-old boys were obese compared to 20% (n=33) of eleven-year-olds. See *Table 3.1* for comparisons.

Table 3.1: Comparisons between nine- and eleven-year-old boys and girls

	Nine-year-old girls	Nine year-old boys	Eleven-year-old girls	Eleven-year-old boys
Overweight	22% (n=56)	22% (n=71)	32% (n=36)	27% (n=41)
Obese	10% (n=27)	10% (n=33)	13% (n=15)	20% (n=33)

In another study, Sahota *et al* (2001a) report that the prevalence of obesity in pre-school children was 6%, rising to 17% by the age of fifteen years. In the same year, Dr Beckie Lang of the Medical Research Centre's Human Nutrition Laboratory was reported in the *Daily Telegraph* (2001b) as stating that in 1980 the prevalence of obese adults in the UK was 6% in men and 8% in women. By 1998, the prevalence was 17% in men and 20% in women. Dr Lang predicted that if the trend continued more than 25% of adults would be obese by 2010. In Ireland, the predicted rate of obesity in 2010 is 23% in women and 22% in men. At present, the average weight for men and women in Ireland is higher than in England, Wales and Scotland (Department of Health, Social Services and Public Safety [DHSSPS], 2002).

There is no consensus in the definition of being overweight or obesity in children. However, the International Obesity Taskforce is cited by Bundred *et al* (2001) who suggest that children over the 80th centile are overweight as this corresponds to a body mass index (BMI) of 25 at the age of eighteen years in both males and females. The BMI is a mathematical formula which is used as a measure of obesity, and is calculated by dividing the body weight (kg) by the square height (m^2). The ideal range for BMI for adults is between 20 and 25 kg/m^2. A person is considered overweight if their BMI is over 25 and obese if it is over 30 (BNF, 2001).

Activity: To calculate your own BMI

1. Take your weight in pounds and multiply that by 704.
2. Divide that number by your height in inches.
3. Divide that number by your height in inches again.

If your score is between 19 and 24.9 it means you are fit.
If your score is between 25 and 29.9 it means you are overweight.
If your score is 30 or more then you are obese.

(Source: http://www.coolnurse.com/dieting.htm)

The primary cause of being overweight or obese is stated to be a sedentary lifestyle and the consumption of energy dense foods (Miles *et al*, 2001). There is evidence that the lay public's perspectives of the causes of obesity differ from general practitioners. Ogden *et al* (2001a) conducted a survey of eighty-nine GPs and 599 patients from practices across the UK. The aim was to compare GPs' and patients' models of obesity. The patients' beliefs about the causes of obesity are shown in *Table 3.2*.

Table 3.2: Causes of obesity

Medical	Genetics/inheritance, glands/hormone problems, slow metabolism
Psychological	Low self-esteem, anxiety/stress, depression
Behavioural	Eating too much, not enough exercise, eating the wrong foods
Social	Unemployment, low income

The GPs were more likely to believe the cause of obesity was over-eating and rated diabetes as an important consequence. Patients believed that their GP and counselling was a solution but GPs believed that the obese person themselves was the most helpful solution. Ogden *et al* (2001b) state that such a model of obesity reflects victim blaming as the person is considered to be responsible for both the cause and the solution.

An additional factor to be considered related to the cause of an increasing overweight and obese population, particularly in children, is the effect of television. The effect of television is twofold. Firstly, sitting watching television reduces the available time for physical activity. Secondly, food advertising on television has an effect. In 1996, Caroli and Lagravinese (2002) noted that food advertising on television occurred mostly during children's television hours and 60% of adverts focused on cereals, confectionery and savoury snacks. Kuribayashi *et al* (2001) assert that the amount of television watched is a good predictor of poor nutritional habits. They believe that the more television is watched, the more likely individuals are to have incorrect conceptions about food and possess incorrect knowledge about nutritional principles. Kuribayashi *et al* (2001) state that television commercials do change behaviour and attitudes including health and nutrition behaviours and as we will see later in this chapter, mass media campaigns are used in this respect to promote healthy eating. However, Kuribayashi *et al* (2001) conclude that both children and adults are watching television commercials that advertise largely unhealthy food.

Consequences of being overweight or obese

A person's diet has a profound influence on their health (Alderson and Ogden, 1999) and there is evidence to link diet with a number of illnesses (Povey *et al*, 2000). The following are attributed to being overweight or obese:

- cardiovascular problems, such as coronary heart disease, hypertension and stroke
- diabetes
- certain cancers
- gallstones
- infertility
- problems in pregnancy.

Miles *et al* (2001) state that obesity is currently one of the most avoidable causes of ill-health, second only to smoking. Obesity and being overweight is associated with a reduction in life expectancy and the development of both physical and psychological conditions, which in turn affect the quality of life (Jeffry, 2001).

Conditions associated with being obese or overweight:

❖ Digestive disorders such as gall-bladder disease.

❖ Respiratory disorders such as dyspnoea and sleep apnoea.

❖ Menstrual abnormalities and hirsutism.

❖ Pregnancy complications: increased risk of neural tube defects, perinatal mortality, hypertension, toxaemia, gestational diabetes, preterm labour, Caesarean section and hospitalisation.

❖ Weight-related musculoskeletal disorders and arthritic diseases.

❖ Stress incontinence.

❖ Psychosocial illness, such as depression, poor self-esteem and diminished social and mental functioning.

❖ Limited mobility and increased fatigue (Jeffry, 2001).

Obese individuals tend to have raised levels of blood cholesterol due to a high intake of saturated fats which are found in cooking fats, butter, lard, fatty meats and meat products, full fat milk, dairy products, chips, biscuits, cakes and confectionery (BNF, 2001). There is evidence that a person's adult health is actually influenced by what they eat as a child. Atherosclerosis development in blood vessels during childhood and research has demonstrated that this is related to the blood cholesterol levels in the child (Alderson and Ogden, 1999).

Being overweight or obese increases the risk of coronary heart disease and the risk is more pronounced if the excess weight is concentrated in the abdominal area. The latter is termed central obesity. BNF (2001) state that it is easier for fat around the waist to have access to the liver's blood supply which in turn decreases the sensitivity of the liver to insulin. In England, 32% of women are overweight (a body mass index [BMI] of $>30kg/m^2$) and 20% are said to have central obesity. Having an unhealthy diet is also a cause of coronary heart disease. Indeed, some 30% of deaths from coronary heart disease are said to be attributable to unhealthy diets and 47% of deaths in women from coronary heart disease are attributable to raised blood cholesterol level (over 5.2mmol/l). The mean blood cholesterol level for women in England is 5.6 mmol/l and some 67% have levels over 5 mmol/l (BHF, 2002).

There is evidence that obesity is a risk factor in the development of gallstones and that rapid loss in such individuals is associated not only with gallstone formation but also gall bladder disease: the warning message is to lose weight gradually and safely (Anon, 1999a). Josefson (2001) reports that obesity and inactivity contribute to up to 33% of cancers of the colon, breast, uterus, kidney and gastro-intestinal tract. There is a theory that being obese and inactive promotes the development of cancer through nutritional and dietary factors.

> *Changes in metabolism and hormonal activity may also be implicated particularly in hormone responsive cancers such as breast and endometrial carcinomas. Oestrogens serve as growth factors for both breast and endometrial cancers and fat cells serve as a source for androtenedione, which is converted into oestrogens.*
>
> (Josepfson, 2001, p. 945)

Rousseau (2001) notes that the increased risk of breast cancer in pre-menopausal women is positively associated with obesity but that the case is less clear between post-menopausal obesity and breast cancer development. Obese or overweight women of childbearing age have an increased risk of infertility and those who do become pregnant, are at greater risk of adverse outcomes (Cogswell *et al*, 2001).

Research indicates that unborn children can be adversely affected by poor nutritional habits of their mothers. For normal foetal growth and development women who are planning to conceive should ensure that they have an adequate intake of folic acid pre-conception and into the first few weeks of pregnancy to promote healthy neural tube development. Pregnant women also require an adequate amount of iron to prevent anaemia and promote normal foetal brain development. Iodine is believed to play a role in later cognitive functioning of the baby and an adequate intake of vitamins A and D helps to ensure normal development of visual and skeletal systems (HDA, 1998). The HDA (1998) state that the birth weight is related to both neonatal and adult health.

A baby, born at full-term weighing more than 2.5kg is more likely to grow up steadily and experience less illnesses than a baby born at a lower weight who is more prone to infections and have difficulties feeding.

Diabetes

It is estimated that there are about 1.3 million people with diagnosed diabetes in the United Kingdom. In 1995 world-wide there was an estimated 135 million people who were diabetic and this figure is predicted to rise to 300 million by 2025. Dyer (2002c) reported the first cases of non-insulin dependent diabetes in white adolescents in the UK, with three thirteen to fifteen-year-old girls and one boy aged fifteen being recently diagnosed. This is alarming as it is well known that the earlier the onset of diabetes is, the higher the rate of complications such as hypertension and blindness occur. Dyer (2002c) reports that obesity rates in children have doubled since 1982 and tripled during that time in adults. With this rising prevalence in obesity, the prediction is that new cases of diabetes will double to 270 million by 2010 and four million of those will be British.

Narayan *et al* (2001) reported their findings from a randomised controlled trial of 522 middle-aged overweight people with impaired glucose tolerance. They found that lifestyle changes could reduce the risk of developing diabetes by 58% over four years. Diabetes substantially increases the risk of coronary heart disease.

It is estimated that nearly 50% of diabetes may be undiagnosed. Women with non-insulin dependent diabetes have between three and fives times the risk of developing coronary heart disease than those who are not diabetic (BHF, 2002). The incidence of diabetes increases with age. The prevalence of diagnosed diabetes has increased by 25% in women since 1991 (BHF, 2002). The rate of non-insulin treated diabetes in women in low socio-economic groups is about 50% higher than those in the more affluent groups. The prevalence of diabetes in Pakistani and Bangladeshi women is fives times greater and four times greater in black Caribbean women than that of the general population. Regular physical activity lowers the risk of developing non-insulin dependent diabetes (Vuori, 1998).

Eating disorders

Eating disorders within young women is a particular public health concern. Cultural pressures on young women are partly attributed to the rise in cases seen in the USA. Lyubomirsky *et al* (2001) report findings from a study involving college women which indicted that

90% had been on slimming diets, two out of every five regularly indulge in full-day fasting and between 50% and 67% admit to binge eating at least occasionally. Nauta *et al* (2001) believe that frequent dieting can contribute to an increased risk of cardiovascular disease. They assert that calorie restriction promotes binge eating and estimate that between 20% and 46% of those requesting treatment for weight problems have a moderate or severe binge-eating problem. According to Nauta *et al* (2001), binge eaters are more vulnerable to depression and have a lower self-esteem than obese individuals who do not indulge in binge eating.

Binge eating is the most common of the eating disorders and involves individuals eating large amounts of food over short periods of time while experiencing a feeling of loss of control. Unlike individuals with bulimia, binge eaters do not vomit or use laxatives after a bingeing episode (Anon, 2001). It is estimated that 1% of women aged between fifteen and thirty are anorexic, 2% have bulimia and 5% will be binge eaters. A smaller but growing number of men are also affected (Mind Out for Mental Health). Irving and Neumark-Sztainer (2002) advise that obese people are more likely to use unhealthy weight losing strategies such as diet pills, self-induced vomiting, laxatives and diuretics. They suggest personal socio-environmental and behavioural approaches are used in an integrated approach to prevention.

Health promotion activities

There is increasing recognition that children are the key individuals to target with healthy eating and physical activity messages. As Wardle and Huon (2000, p. 39) state:

> *The promotion of healthier eating patterns among children is considered to be a priority in view of the mounting evidence for 'tracking' both of food choices and risk factors which indicates that children with poor diets are likely to become adults with poor diets.*

Povey *et al* (2000) remark that healthy eating is often construed as being virtuous but not enjoyable and they attribute this to childhood experiences and being told to eat certain foods up as they are 'good for you'.

Children and adolescents who are overweight or obese are likely to be overweight or obese in their adulthood, as habitual eating behaviours adopted in childhood are difficult to change in later life (Caroli and Lagravinese, 2002). Furthermore, mothers who are prone to overeating are more likely to have overweight children, especially girls, which gives credence to the assertion that overeating is in part a learned behaviour (Anon, 1999b). Dowdra *et al* (2001) report that children in families with one or two overweight parents consume a higher percentage of their energy intake as fat and they believe that this contributes to the development of overweight children.

Sahota *et al* (2001a) conducted a randomised controlled trial to assess if a school-based intervention was effective in reducing the risk factors for obesity. Their sample was 634 children between the ages of seven and eleven years. Following implementation of the health promotion programme, they found positive changes in classroom health education and school food service (Sahota *et al*, 2001b). Having such an educational intervention programme increased the children's exposure to healthy eating messages and increased their knowledge, but Sahota *et al* (2001a) were disappointed that children demonstrated minimal behavioural changes although there was a modest increase in their consumption of vegetables.

Atkinson and Nitzke (2001) comment on Sahota *et al*'s work and make the conclusion that in order to have the most cost-effective action, the programmes should be targeted at high-risk children and devote resources in this way. However, the danger, as they remark, is that by targeting high-risk children, there is the potential to produce more stigmatisation which in turn can lead to the child developing an eating disorder. Atkinson and Nitzke (2001) recommend that more research is conducted to identify the most appropriate strategies to use in the treatment of obesity in children.

Dixey *et al* (2001a) conducted qualitative focus groups with 300 children aged between nine and eleven years with the aim of exploring the children's perceptions of a healthy diet, the links between diet and health and what they thought influenced their eating behaviour. They found that most groups understood the concept of a well-balanced diet and the importance of eating in moderation. Dixey *et al* report that children spontaneously linked the concept of thinness and fatness to concepts of healthy eating. There was an understanding that a food that was considered healthy was good for them and not fattening. When asked what they thought the health consequences of an unhealthy diet were, the majority view was arterial disease and heart problems.

The second most commonly cited consequence was becoming too fat, the inability to move and take part in sports. When the researchers explored with the children their perceptions of thinness and fatness, they found that children had a good concept of the dangers of being too thin and they had appropriate understanding of eating disorders. Girls more than boys voiced social concerns about being too fat and both genders believed that fat people were more likely to get bullied. There were many factors that influenced these children in what they ate, including advertising, parents, home environment, and pocket money. Dixey *et al* (2001b) conclude that to change children's behaviour in terms of what they eat, it is imperative to gain their active participation and not to resort to coercion as children would find ways around eating what they enjoy.

Alderson and Ogden (1999) reported from studies which indicated that children will select different foods when they are being watched by their parents compared to when they are not. They also report that children tend to want to eat the foods that they have been given the most and prefer what is acceptable and available in their household. Rather worryingly, Alderson and Ogden suggest that mothers who are dieting may restrain their own food intake by feeding their children some of the foods that they themselves are forbidden.

With respect to the participation of children in a healthy eating promotional campaign, Baranowski *et al* (2002) conducted a randomised controlled trial to evaluate the effectiveness of a school nutrition education programme based on social cognition theory. The programme was called 'Gimme 5' and the researchers used a variety of mediums to spread the message: curriculum; newsletters; videotapes; point of purchase education and rewards. The rewards involved children being awarded points for dietary changes and the points could be exchanged for prizes. The whole programme was designed to be fun and participatory while targeting behavioural change and encouraging the daily intake of five portions of fruit and vegetables. Their findings demonstrated improvement in the consumption of fruit and vegetables, and related psychosocial behaviour and knowledge.

The Government's Committee on the Medical Aspects of Food and Nutrition Policy (COMA) made recommendations in 1994, which specified a number of measures to improve our diet. These measures included reducing our saturated fat and salt intake and increasing carbohydrate, fruit and vegetable consumption.

Kant *et al* (2000) report that a diet containing fruit, vegetables, whole grains and low in dairy fat and lean meat lowers the mortality risk. It is now commonly quoted that we should all eat at least five portions of fruit and vegetables every day. The rationale behind this recommendation is that this amount boosts the body's stores of antioxidant nutrients (Broekmans *et al*, 2000). Antioxidants are thought to inhibit the development of atherosclerosis and are also found in tea, red wine, apples and onions (Wood *et al*, 1998). Fruit and vegetables are also rich sources of potassium, which is associated with lower blood pressure and risk of stroke (*Coronary Heart Disease: Guidance for implementing the preventive aspects of the National Service Framework*). Government recommendations also suggest that we should reduce our intake of salt by one third as this can lower blood pressure and prevent the increase of blood pressure with age (Wood *et al*, 1998).

One reason why fresh fruit and vegetables reduce the risk of coronary heart disease may be due to the presence of salicylic acid which is the anti-inflammatory agent found in aspirin. Researchers have found that the salicylic acid levels in the blood of vegetarians are twelve times higher than those who have a normal diet. The benefits are perceived to be due to the anti-inflammatory properties of salicylic acid which reduces the hardening and narrowing of arteries (Health Media News, 2001).

The National Diet and Nutrition survey found that while the eating of fresh fruit has increased fourfold since the 1940s, the intake of fresh vegetables has decreased. Moreover, the survey indicated that only 19% of girls in the two to fifteen age group eat fruit more than once a day. Wardle (1995) cited by Alderson and Ogden (1999) found that children between nine and eleven years of age continued to have an inadequate intake of fruit and vegetables, consuming less than 50% of the recommended levels. Only 5% exceeded the recommended levels. In 2001, BBC News Online reported that a MORI poll had discovered that as many as 200,000 children in England and Wales had not eaten any fruit or vegetables in the previous week. The poll found that, on average, children were eating less than thirteen portions of fruit and vegetables a week compared to the recommended guidelines of at least thirty-five portions a week.

In the Scottish Health Education Population Survey of 1998, it was found that 39% of respondents did not eat fruit or vegetables daily and 36% were unable to cite the recommended levels. The least likely group to eat fruit and vegetables were young men. Eighty-three per cent of the respondents stated that they had tried to make at least one change in their diet in the past year. This was broken down into the following areas:

- eating more fruit and vegetables (47%)
- eating less fatty foods (41%)
- using low fat alternatives (38%)
- eating less sugary foods (36%).

Bangladeshi women eat more red meat and fried foods and less fruit than men do in other ethnic groups. However, Indian women are less likely to eat red meat or fried foods. Chinese women have the highest fruit and vegetable consumption compared to women from other ethnic groups. The lowest level of vegetable consumption is among the Pakistani community (BNF, 2001).

Wardle and Huon (2000) state that fewer than 15% of the UK population adhere to the recommended limitations on consuming saturated fat. *The Coronary Heart Disease: Guidance for implementing the preventive aspects of the National Service Framework* remarks that the most striking difference between groups of individuals in the UK, is that those in lower socio-economic groups have a tendency to eat about one third less fruit and vegetables than those in higher socio-economic groups. This difference is also noted in children.

The reduction in the amount of fat in the diet, particularly saturated fat, is aimed at reducing health risks. A 10% reduction in saturated fat intake is related to a corresponding reduction effect of 20% to 30% in coronary heart disease mortality (*Coronary Heart Disease: Guidance for implementing the preventive aspects of the National Service Framework*).

Parmenter *et al* (2000) conducted a survey of 1040 individuals to examine the nutrition knowledge and demographic variations in knowledge, in a wide cross-section of adults in England. The first section of the questionnaire related to dietary recommendations. Results indicated that more than 90% were aware of recommendations to reduce intake of fat, sugar and salt and increase fruit, vegetables and fibre. However, there were a number unaware of other recommendations, such as to reduce intake of saturated fat (25%); to reduce intake of meat (51%) and to eat more starchy carbohydrates (90%). Furthermore, 70% could not state the recommended daily intake of fruit and vegetables and just over 50% thought that three portions a day was adequate.

Knowledge related to food groups was the second section. Findings revealed that their knowledge about fibre was satisfactory but about 50% were unaware that cheese was high in salt, and the majority had poor knowledge about monounsaturated fat with less than 2% knowing that olive oil contains mostly this type of fat.

The section on diet and disease relationships revealed that almost 15% were unaware of the link between a high fat intake and disease but those that were aware of the link knew it could cause heart disease. Parmenter *et al* (2000) report that 41% of the survey sample were unaware of the consequences of developing health problems and a low intake of fruit and vegetables.

Only 42% knew that eating more fruit and vegetables can help to reduce the risk of cancer and 47% knew it could also reduce the risk of coronary heart disease. The link between a high salt intake and cardiovascular problems was identified by 84%. Most of the sample thought that sugar could cause diabetes and obesity but only about 25% mentioned tooth decay. The poorest item in this section was that only 22% of respondents had ever heard of anti-oxidants. Women had a slightly greater level of knowledge than men did. And it was noted that those in the youngest age group scored lower than those in middle years, with those aged over sixty-five obtaining the lowest scores. Finally, individuals who were married or living together achieved slightly higher scores than those who were either single, separated, divorced or widowed (Parmenter *et al*, 2000).

There are a number of barriers associated with eating a healthier diet. A population survey found lack of will power was identified by 35%, followed by health foods being too expensive (25%), not liking the taste of healthy foods (15%), and not knowing what changes to make (15%).

Men most commonly cited the latter two barriers. Related to will power is self-efficacy which relates to the person's perceptions of whether they will achieve their goal or not. If they believe that attaining the goal will be relatively easy and that they will have a degree of control over the change in their behaviour then they are more likely to succeed (Povey *et al*, 2000). For this reason, Povey *et al* suggest that health promotion strategies that aim to promote health-related changes in diet would benefit by targeting people's attitudes and their self-efficacy over the change.

Parmenter *et al* (2000) offer some additional suggestions to overcome barriers: fruit and vegetables are inexpensive if bought in season; eat fruit as snacks, on top of cereal, and making healthy eating fun for children, for example, using vegetables with dips.

According to the DoH (1999), a 10% reduction in cholesterol lowers the risk of coronary heart disease by 50% at age forty and 20% at seventy. Eating oily fish also contributes to a reduction in risk of developing coronary heart disease as oily fish contains polyunsaturated fatty acids which reduces blood viscosity and inhibits clot formation (BNF, 2001). A sustained weight loss of between five and ten kilograms (11–22lbs) could reduce the chances of fatal coronary heart disease by 9%, and could reduce the risk of cancer by more than 30% (DHSSPS, 2002).

In order to change people's nutritional behaviour, there has to be some sort of stimulus to make the change. Good intentions are not enough. Parmenter *et al* (2002) found that a catalyst was the perception of or experience of actual health problems or illness. Koikkalainen *et al* (2002) found that more than 60% of individuals report that as a result of experiencing a myocardial infarction, they have made changes to their dietary intake by avoiding fast foods, confectionery and cakes. Their weight has reduced and they tend to have less frequent relapses than they did in the past.

> *Obesity cannot be prevented or managed, nor physical activity promoted, solely at the level of individual governments, the food industry, international agencies, the media, communities, and individuals all need to work together to modify the environment so that it is less conducive to weight gain.*

(Josefson, 2001, citing WHO panel, p. 945)

Using available evidence, the *Coronary Heart Disease: Guidance for implementing the preventive aspects of the National Service Framework* suggest the following to achieve effective intervention:

* Focus on diet alone or diet plus physical activity rather than tackling a range of factors.

* Set clear goals, based on theories of behavioural change, rather than relying on the provision of information alone.

* Include personal contact with individuals or small groups sustained over time.

* Provide personal feedback on any changes in behaviour and risk factors.

* Promote changes in the local environments, for example, in shops and catering outlets to help people choose a healthy diet.

They conclude that providing information is insufficient alone but that a combination of information and development of skills to implement knowledge into actual practice is more effective.

The *Coronary Heart Disease: Guidance for implementing the*

preventive aspects of the National Health Service Framework suggests features of effective interventions in school and workplace strategies (*Table 3.3*).

Table 3.3: Effective features of interventions in school and the workplace

School interventions	Workplace interventions
Nutrition education interventions are more likely to be effective when they employ educational strategies that are directly relevant to a particular behaviour (eg. diet or physical activity) and are derived from appropriate theory and research	Visible and enthusiastic support and involvement from management
	Involvement by employees at all levels in the planning and implementation phases
Interventions need adequate time and intensity to be effective	A focus on definable and modifiable risk factors rather than multiple risk factor interventions
Family involvement enhances the effectiveness of programmes for younger children	Screening and/or individual counselling
Incorporation of self-evaluation or self-assessment and feedback is effective for older children	Changes to the composition of best selling foods provided in canteens and vending machines
Effective nutrition education includes consideration of the whole school environment and community	Tailoring to the characteristics and needs of employees
Interventions in the larger community can enhance school nutrition education	Use of local resources in organisation and implementation of the intervention
The most effective interventions focus on diet alone or diet and physical activity	Combine population-based policy initiatives with intensive individual and group-orientated interventions
	Built in sustainability

In 1999, the USA produced unitary diet guidelines with the intention that six simple, easy to remember rules would be applicable to all except those under the age of two years. The six rules are:

1.   Eat a variety of foods.
2.   Choose most foods from plant sources.
3.   Eat five or more servings of fruit and vegetables each day.
4.   Eat six or more servings of bread, cereals, pasta and/or rice each day.

5.   Eat high fat foods sparingly, particularly those from animal sources.
6.   Keep intake of simple sugars to a minimum.

With these six rules, the intention is for fat consumption to be no more than 30% of calorie intake, saturated fat being less than 10%, salt intake about one level teaspoon a day and cholesterol, limited to 300mgs a day (Tanne, 1999).

Using the media

The BBC programme 'Fighting Fat, Fighting Fit' was launched in 1999 and was the largest ever health education campaign which ran over seven weeks and had prime time slots during the day and evening, both on television and radio (Miles *et al*, 2001). The aim was explicitly to get people to lose weight by exercising and eating healthily. It emphasised that small incremental and lasting changes to one's lifestyle were more beneficial than aiming for rapid and short-term results. The programme became part of a research study in which 6000 people were randomly selected to take part. The programme was found to be highly popular and it was estimated that 75% of the UK population were aware of it. At follow-up, five months later, it was found that individuals' intake of fruit and vegetables was higher, fatty foods and snack intake was lower, there were positive changes to psychological well-being and an increase in activity (Miles *et al*, 2001). Despite many people being aware of this programme, only 1% of the population are thought to have participated in it (Wardle *et al*, 2001). It was noticeable that men under the age of twenty-five did not take part in the campaign and therefore, Miles *et al* (2001) suggest that this group require specific targeting.

Mercer and Tessier (2001) state that most general practitioners and practice nurses favour their overweight or obese patients attending commercial slimming clubs. These clubs normally have programmes which include behavioural, dietary and exercise components and have been found to be effective (Cioffi, 2002).

Physical activity

> *When you rest, you rust.*
>
> (Martin Luther)

> *It has been suspected since the 1950s that physical inactivity increases the risk of developing CHD (Coronary Heart Disease), but it was not until the 1990s that sufficient evidence had accumulated to justify including physical inactivity among the major risk factors for CHD. Physical inactivity is now also considered an established risk factor for Type 2 diabetes, obesity and hypertension.*
>
> (European Heart Network, 1999, cited by BHF, 2001)

It is thought-provoking to reflect that 37% of deaths from coronary heart disease are attributed to physical inactivity compared with 19% attributed to smoking (BHF, 2001).

Sparling *et al* (2000) remind us that the human species was designed for movement and that our bodies have an inherent need to be exercised. Carnall (2000) refers to the inherent need for the human body to exercise and bemoans our increasingly motorised existence. He states that we now walk, on average, eight miles less a day than our forebears fifty years ago and provides other thought-provoking statistics such as:

- in 1949, 34% of miles were travelled by bicycle whereas today only 1–2% are
- seventy per cent of all trips made by car are five miles or less in length and alternative means such as cycling or walking could be used
- today, 70% of the British population participate in any form of physical activity less than once a month.

Weist and Lyle (1997) believe it is important that the terms physical activity, exercise and physical fitness are differentiated between in order that healthcare professionals can use the most appropriate terminology. According to Weist and Lyle (1997, p. 11), physical activity denotes:

> *... any bodily movement produced by skeletal muscles that result in energy expenditure. Exercise is a subset of physical activity and can be defined as a planned, structured and*

repetitive bodily movement done to improve or maintain one or more components of physical fitness. Physical fitness is a set of attributes that people have or achieve that relates to the ability to perform physical activity.

The terms vigorous and moderate exercise are often used in recommendations related to physical activity but they are rarely defined. The Exercise Alliance (2001) provides the following information:

Vigorous physical activity is any activity which makes the heart beat rapidly and breathing fairly hard (but not breathless) and may make the individual perspire (but not profusely). Vigorous activity relates to the 'old' (but still valid) 3 x 20 minutes of exercise per week message and is associated more with structured exercise or competitive sports. Typical activities would include: running, jogging, squash, swimming hard, cycling, basketball, football, and aerobics. Vigorous activity provides fitness and health benefits with the same emphasis on fitness. Health benefits are about the same as for 'moderate' activity.

Moderate physical activity is any activity which makes the breathing slightly harder than normal and the person feel warmer (but not perspiring). Moderate activity relates to the 'new' 5 x up to 30 minutes of activity a week message. Activity can be accumulated in ten- to fifteen-minute chunks to achieve thirty minutes in a day. This message is more associated with unstructured activity, which can be more easily fitted into daily routine. Typical examples include: brisk walking; slow swimming; heavy gardening (digging, mowing); heavy housework (washing floors, windows); tennis; badminton; line dancing and light aerobics. Moderate activity focuses on the health benefits (prevention of disease etc.) which are about the same as for vigorous activity. Fitness gains are not as great as for vigorous activity.

There are many health benefits ascribed to taking regular exercise. The Exercise Alliance (2001) lists the benefits of physical exercise as:

Physical

- reduces risk of coronary heart disease
- reduces risk of stroke

- helps with weight maintenance and weight control
- prevention and management of osteoporosis
- prevention and control of high blood pressure
- reduces cholesterol levels
- helps prevent and improve non-insulin dependent diabetes
- maintains flexibility, strength and functional capacity
- reduces stress and anxiety
- reduces mild depression
- reduces risk of cancer of the colon
- potentially reduces healthcare cost.

Psychosocial

- reduces stress
- relieves symptoms of depression, anxiety and mood
- raises self-esteem.

Economic

- the costs of coronary heart disease to the NHS and social care system were estimated to be £1,630 million in 1996
- it is estimated that 9% of coronary heart disease could be avoided if physical activity was increased
- potentially this means a saving of £144 million to the healthcare system.

Vuori (1998) asserts that many of the above effects disappear within two and eight months if the physical activity is not maintained. Vuori (1998) states that regular physical activity is associated with a decreased risk of colon cancer but that there is no association with rectal cancer. The risk of cancer of the colon in the physically active is between 20% and 50% lower than their sedentary counterparts. Vuori also states that there may be some evidence to suggest that physical activity may play a part in reducing the risk of developing breast or prostate cancer.

There is a positive association between physical activity and mood and a general feeling of well being. Exercising produces more energy and has the effect of making one think more clearly and improves sleeping patterns (Teitz, 2000). A number of authors note the positive effect that physical activity and exercise can have on chronic health conditions. It will help ameliorate the pain associated with arthritis; reduce the risk of coronary heart disease, diabetes, and depression as well as reducing cognitive decline (Deuster, 1996; Gill *et al*, 1997; Teitz, 2000; Hunt *et al*, 2001). Women who have diabetes and coronary heart disease have a four to six times greater risk of mortality than women who are not diabetic. The figure for men is two to three times greater. The reason for this increased risk is unknown (Woods and Mitchell, 1997).

Women who walk briskly or exercise vigorously for three hours every week reduce their risk of developing coronary heart disease (Manson *et al*, 1999). Regular aerobic exercise helps to reduce the risk of developing coronary heart disease as it prevents or slows down the laying down of atherosclerotic plaque in blood vessels (Woolf-May *et al*, 1999). Haapanen *et al* (1997) suggest that physical activity has a preventative effect not only on coronary heart disease, but also on hypertension and diabetes. The British Heart Foundation (2002) estimates that 38% of deaths from coronary heart disease are due to a lack of exercise.

The Exercise Alliance (2001) argues that since 65% of people in the UK are sedentary compared to only 28% who smoke, increasing physical activity will have a greater potential heart health gain than stopping smoking. Imagine the dual benefits! The Exercise Alliance (2001) also reports that the fitter you are the less likely you are to die and cite research which demonstrates an average longevity increase of nine years in high fit individuals and seven years in medium fit compared to sedentary individuals. Fitter individuals are 70% less likely to develop mobility problems, which can threaten one's independence. Vuori (1998) suggests that the effect on mortality is largely due to aerobic and endurance activity.

Haapanien *et al* (1997) report that a sedentary lifestyle in women was more likely to increase their risk of developing diabetes than coronary heart disease or hypertension. Less active men and women are estimated to be at 30% greater risk of developing hypertension than their most active counterparts.

The likelihood of females developing dementia or cognitive impairment is reduced by 50% in those with a high level of physical activity and the risk of Alzheimer's disease in the same group is reduced by up to 70% (Anon, 2001).

Despite the obvious benefits of physical exercise, only small proportions of us participate in the recommended levels. Romans (1997) states that approximately 27% of American women achieved the recommended levels while the remainder are sedentary or exercise irregularly. Hunt *et al* (2001) provide the following figures for the UK:

- the least active amongst us are nearly twice as likely to suffer from coronary heart disease
- the risk of inactivity is similar to that of cigarette smoking, obesity, hypertension and high cholesterol levels
- Seventy per cent of men and 80% of women do not reach the recommended levels of exercising three times per week for a minimum of twenty minutes duration.

Deuster (1996) adds that between the ages of eighteen and thirty-seven, women may decrease their physical activity by as much as 50%. This is reinforced by Ferron *et al* (1999). It is estimated that 25% of women in the UK do not participate in any sustained exercise (Wyn and Solis, 2001).

The Exercise Alliance (2001) provides participation rates of physical activity among people from black and minority ethnic groups. Among African-Caribbean's aged between sixteen and seventy-four, 32% of men and 31% of women are sedentary compared with 24% of the general population. Activity levels among South Asian women aged between sixteen and seventy-four vary: 83% of Indians, 86% of Pakistanis and 82% of Bangladeshis do not take part in enough physical activity to benefit their health, compared to 68% of women in the general population.

The implications of this inactivity are addressed by the Exercise Alliance (2001) who state that 30% of men and 60% of women cannot maintain a speed of three miles per hour when walking up a moderate slope. This includes most men over fifty-five years of age and women over thirty-five years of age. Furthermore, 55% of women aged between fifty-five and sixty-five years and 30% of men in the age group sixty-five to seventy-four years are below the functional threshold for knee strength. The latter is required to get out of a chair unaided.

The recommendation is to exercise aerobically for at least thirty minutes, five days a week. Apparently, only 25% of women in the UK meet this recommendation. It is recommended that children (five to eighteen years) undertake some form of moderate exercise for at least one hour per day.

In England, it is reported that 39% of girls meet this target. By the time girls are fifteen years old the rate of activity drops with only 18% of girls reaching the recommended target. Seven out of ten women are not physically active enough to benefit their health (DoH, 1999). In 2001, the British Heart Foundation recommended that the message should be that to improve health and help with weight management, adults should try to build up gradually to accumulate half-an-hour of moderately intense physical activity on five or more days of the week. Activities such as brisk walking, cycling, swimming, dancing and gardening are considered to be the most appropriate. As the British Heart Foundation (2001) point out, the new message emphasises the aim for overall health gains rather than only confined to cardiovascular fitness. This recommendation makes a departure from previous recommendations (twenty minutes vigorous and structured activity three times a week) (BHF, 2001). The following points are offered by the BHF (2001) as being the advantages and disadvantages of the new message:

Advantages

❖ It is a safer message and more achievable for most people.

❖ For those who are very inactive, accumulating energy expenditure at a relatively low level of intensity is more feasible and is less likely to result in lapse of activity.

❖ At a lower intensity, individuals are able to exercise for longer and thereby achieve a greater total energy expenditure than would result from shorter, more intensive bouts of activity.

❖ New message is more manageable, accommodating daily activities as well as formal exercise.

❖ Moderate intensity exercise is easier and more enjoyable to perform.

Disadvantages

❖ Not a specific message and therefore more difficult to promote than the previous message.

❖ It is a very soft message — doesn't seem enough.

❖ Difficult to quantify moderate exercise — doctors and patients don't like doing things they cannot measure.

According to Bennett and Murphy (1997), individuals who expend more than 2000 kcals of energy in exercise activities per week live on average 2.5 years longer than those who do not. Those who engage in exercise are more likely to be young, male, well educated and in a high socio-economic group. The least likely individuals to exercise are older, belong to lower socio-economic groups and their health is likely to be at risk as a consequence of smoking and being overweight or obese (Bennett and Murphy, 1997).

Just as nutritional patterns are established in childhood, physical exercise or the lack of it can influence activity patterns in adulthood. In a 1989 study of physical activity in ten- to thirteen-year-old Irish children, it was found that only a third of the sample exercised four or more times a week. Only 23% walked or cycled to school. By 1998, 53% of nine- to seventeen-year-old Irish children exercised four times or more per week. It was noticeable that boys tended to exercise more than girls (Hussey *et al*, 2001).

In their 2001 study, Hussey *et al* found that 39% of children participated in hard exercise for at least twenty minutes three or more times a week and they concluded that it was concerning that 25% of girls and 14% of boys were exercising less than the minimum recommendations. Additionally, they found that 33% of children were driven to school by car and 5% by bus. Some 40% walked to school and 20% walked part of the way. In their previous study in 1999, some 71% had been driven to school so the recent figures indicate an improvement.

> *Motivation is at the crux of health behaviour performance and thus, to a great extent, health (and it can be defined as) the intrinsic determination toward goal attainment of exercise adherence among psychological variables studied.*
>
> (Plonczynski, 2000, p. 695)

Motivation plays the largest role in adherence to physical activity. Factors associated with motivation are the desire for health maintenance and fitness. Barriers to motivation are a perceived lack of time and threat of pain and musculoskeletal problems (Teitz, 2000), and lack of support from family and friends and perceived incapacity due to ageing (Bennett and Murphy, 1997). Garber (1997) suggests that 50% of men and women who take up exercise will drop out within six months. Lack of time is the most commonly cited barrier to taking more exercise. Perceived barriers to physical activity for black and ethnic minorities are shared with those of the general population but there are additional cultural and religious issues which affect the manner of participation, for example, single gender provision and dress codes for South Asian people (Exercise Alliance, 2001).

The British Heart Foundation (2001) provide the following suggestions to help overcome barriers to activity (*Table 3.4*).

Table 3.4: Suggestions to overcome barriers to activity

Barrier	Solution
Lack of knowledge and information	Provide leaflets/education
Lack of time often due to other priorities	Now recognised benefits through accumulation
Lack of exercise partner/social support	Check out community schemes
Not the 'sporty' type	Refer to 'activity', not sport/exercise
Financial constraints	Walking — best activity, free
Lack of available facilities	Facilities are not always necessary
Lack of motivation and will power	Present the evidence of the benefits of activity/risks of inactivity
Fear of injury, fear of embarrassment	Walking is the safest activity
Don't enjoy it	Variety of activities — hopefully, find something
Fear of doing too much activity	Start very slowly and gradually build up current levels of activity

To maintain a regimen of exercise, requires it to be tied in with daily activities and enjoyment. The Health Education Board for Scotland (HEBS) came up with a slogan 'Hassle-free Exercise' for their campaign in 1995. The ability to incorporate exercise into one's daily routine and exercising at home have been identified as influencing factors in maintaining physical activity (Garber, 1997). The Health Education Board for Scotland (2000) emphasises a small increase in physical activity at all levels, which is incorporated into the daily routine thereby increasing the likelihood that the change is sustainable.

Hunt *et al* (2001) point out that the maximum benefit accrued from physical activity is in the middle-age years as it is then that there is a marked increase in the prevalence of coronary heart disease morbidity and mortality.

The DoH (2001) recommended levels are thirty minutes of moderate exercise five times a week. By not achieving this, the DoH (2001) state that individuals are at twice the risk of coronary heart disease and three times the risk of developing a stroke. Unfortunately, as Coleman and Hendry (1999) report, despite the knowledge that long-term physical activity is associated with a reduction in the risk of coronary heart disease, it appears to be an insufficient impetus for commencing physical activity in young people. It is pertinent to note that those young people who possess a high personal value are more likely to take care of themselves and exercise. Ferron *et al* (1999) and Dowdra *et al* (2001) suggest that in such young people, sport and exercise may be a protective factor against the use of tobacco and drugs as the incidence of their use is low in this group of individuals.

The Health Education Authority (1998) provides the following recommendations and physical activity for young people (five to eighteen-year-olds) (*Table 3.5*).

Strength training is not only important in young people, but also in the elderly as it has been shown to improve balance. Improvement in balance is believed to reduce the incidence of falls in the elderly as epidemiological studies consistently associate physical activity (both past and current) with protection against hip fractures, reducing the risk by up to 50% (Bahr, 2001). It is well recognised that half of those who suffer a fractured hip do not regain their previous physical or functional ability prior to their fall and, consequently, lose their independence: a common reason for admission into long-term care facilities (DHSSPS, 2001).

Incorporating physical activity into everyday behaviours is a complex issue (Miilunpalo *et al*, 2000). Benefits of aerobic exercise can be derived from walking and fitness and health benefits can be gained from moderate intensity exercise accumulated in fifteen-minute bouts during the day (Woolf-May *et al*, 1999). The successful promotion of physical activity requires a multi-disciplinary approach (Sparling *et al*, 2000).

Table 3.5: Recommendations for young people

Recommendations	Rationale	Examples/suggested activities
All young people should participate in physical activity (PA) or at least moderate activity for one hour per day	Most young people are currently doing thirty minutes of moderate PA per day on most days	Brisk walking, cycling, swimming, most sports, dance
Young people who currently do little activity should participate in PA of at least moderate intensity for half-an-hour per day	Childhood overweight and obesity is increasing	Carried out as part of transportation, physical education, games, sport, recreation, work or structured exercise or for younger children as part of active play
At least twice a week, some of these activities should help to enhance and maintain muscular strength and flexibility and bone health	Many young people possess at least one modifiable risk factor	Performed in a continuous fashion or accumulated throughout the day
	Many young people have symptoms of psychological distress	Strength enhancing activities: play (climbing, skipping, jumping), structured exercise (body conditioning, resistance exercises)
	Participation in strength and weight-bearing activities is positively associated with bone mineral density and can be related to reduced risk of osteoporosis	Weight bearing activities; gymnastics, dance, aerobics, skipping and sports such as basketball
	Muscular strength is required to perform activities of daily life (eg. lifting, carrying, bending, twisting)	
	Trunk strength and muscular flexibility may be associated with reduced risk of back pain in later life	

(Source: Cale and Harris, 2001)

Suggested web resources

http://www.bda.uk.com The website of the British Diabetic Association

http://www.defra.gov.uk Ministry of Agriculture, Fisheries and Food website

http://ww.diabetes.org.uk

http://www.edauk.com Eating disorders Association

http://www.hsis.org Since its launch in 1999 HSIS has become a valuable information source for the media, providing up-to-date, factual information about vitamins, minerals and food supplements with the backing of an Advisory Panel made up of independent experts including dieticians, medical experts, GPs and other specialists.

http://www.medicine-chest.co.uk PAGB has produced this site to complement the HSIS site

http://www.hebs.scot.nhs.uk/learningcentre/weightmanagement This is an educational resource for primary health care professionals. The programme is free, but it does require users to register first

http://www.nutsoc.org.uk The website of the Nutrition Society which contains information on scientific information on nutrition and its application to human and animal health

http://show.scot.nhs.uk/diabetes A major new website for information about diabetes in Scotland launched in Spring 2002

http://www.wellbeing.com/index.jsp The Boots website has a large, well written section on vitamins and minerals

http://www.whi.org.uk Walking the Way to Health Initiative

References

Alderson TS, Ogden J (1999) What do mothers feed their children and why? *Health Educ Res* **14**(6): 717–27

Anon (1999a) Weight patterns and cholesytectomy risk. *Women's Health in Primary Care* **2**(9) 702

Anon (1999b) Women who overeat 'teach' their daughters to do the same. *Women's Health in Primary Care* **2**(11): 862

Anon (2001) Exercise helps prevent cognitive decline. *Women's Health in Primary Care* **4**(11): 722

Atkinson RL, Nitzke SA (2001) School based programmes on obesity. *Br Med J* **323**:1018–9

Bahr R (2001) Sports medicine. *Br Med J* **323**: 328–31

Baranowski T, Davis M, Resnicow K (2000) Gimme 5 fruit, juice, and vegetables for fun and health: outcome evaluation. *Health Educ Behav* **27**: 96–111

BBC News Online (2001) *Children's diets lacking in fruit and vegetables* 16/11/01. http://www.bbc.co.uk (accessed January 2002)

Bennett P, Murphy S (1997) *Psychology and Health Promotion*. Open University Press, Aylesbury

British Heart Foundation (2001) *Physical Activity Toolkit: a training pack for primary health care teams*. British Heart Foundation

British Heart Foundation (BHF) (2002) *Coronary Heart Disease Statistics*. http://www.dphpc.ox.uk/bhfhprg/stats/2000/2002/keyfacts/index.html (accessed February 2002)

British Nutrition Foundation (BNF) (2001) *Coronary Heart Disease*. http://www.nutrition.org.uk (accessed February 2002)

Broekmans W Klopping-Ketelaars, I, Schuurman C (2000) Fruits and vegetables increase plasma carotenoids and vitamins and decrease homocysteine in humans. *J Nutr* **130**: 1578–83

Bundred P, Kitchiner D, Buchan I (2001) Prevalence of overweight and obese children between 1989 and 1998: population-based series of cross-sectional studies. *Br Med J* **322**: 1–4

Cale L, Harris J (2001) Exercise recommendations for young people: an update. *Health Educ* **10**(3):126–38

Carnall D (2000) Cycling and health promotion. *Br Med J* **320**: 888

Caroli M, Lagravinese D (2002) Prevention of obesity. *Nutr Res* **22**: 221–6

Cioffi J (2002) Clients' experience of a weight management programme: a qualitative study. *Health Educ* **102**(1): 16–22

Cogswell ME, Perry GS, Schieve LA, Dietz WH (2001) Obesity in women of childbearing age: risks, prevention and treatment. *Primary Care Update Ob/Gyns* **8**(3): 89–105

Coleman JC, Hendry LB (1999) *The Nature of Adolescence*. 3rd edn. Routledge, London

Committee on the Medical Aspects of Food and Nutrition Policy (COMA) 1994

Department of Health (1999) *Saving Lives: Our Healthier Nation*. DoH, London

Department of Health (2001) *The Annual Report of the Chief Medical Officer of the Department of Health 2001: On the State of the Public Health*. DoH, London

Department of Health, Social Services and Public Safety (2002) *Investing for Health*. http://www.dhsspsni.gov.uk/publications/ (accessed February 2002)

Deuster PA (1996) Exercise in the prevention and treatment of chronic disorders. *Women's Health Issues* **6**(6): 320–31

Dixey R, Sahota P, Atwal S, Turner A (2001a) 'Ha ha, you're fat, we're strong'; a qualitative study of boys' and girls' perceptions of fatness, thinness, social pressures and health using focus groups. *Health Educ* **101**(5): 206–16

Dixey R, Sahota P, Atwal S, Turner A (2001b) Children talking about healthy eating: data from focus groups with 300 nine- to eleven-year olds. *British Nutrition Foundation Nutrition Bulletin* **26**: 71–9

Dowdra M, Ai BE, Addy CL, Saunders R, Riner W (2001) Environmental influences, physical activity, and weight status in 8- to 16-year-olds. *Arch Pediatr Adolesc Med* **155**: 711–17

Dyer O (2002) First cases of type 2 diabetes found in UK teenagers. *Br Med J* **324**: 506

European Heart Network (1999) *Physical Activity and Cardiovascular Disease Prevention in the European Union*. Brussels

Exercise Alliance (2001) http://www.exercisealliance.org.uk (accessed February 2002)

Ferron C, Narring F, Cauderay M, Michaud PA (1999) Sport activity in adolescence: associations with health perceptions and experimental behaviours. *Health Educ Res* **14**(2): 225–33

Garber CE (1997) The benefits of physical activity on coronary heart disease and coronary heart disease risk factors in women. *Women's Health Issues* **7**(1): 17–23

Gill DL, Williams K, Williams L, Butki BD, Kim BJ (1997) Physical activity and psychological well-being in older women. *Women's Health Issues* **7**(1): 3–9

Haapanien N, Miilunpalo S, Vuori I, Oja P, Pasanen M (1997) Association of leisure time physical activity with the risk of coronary heart disease, hypertension and diabetes in middle-aged men and women. *Int J Epidemiol* **26**(4): 739–47

Health Development Agency (1998) Effectiveness of interventions to promote healthy eating in pregnant women and women of childbearing age. *Health promotion effectiveness reviews Summary Bulletin 11*. http://www/hda-online.org.uk/html/research/effectivenessreviews/erereview11html (accessed January 2002)

Health Development Agency *Coronary Heart Disease: Guidance for implementing the preventative aspects of the National Service Framework*. HDA, London

Health Education Agency (1998) *Young and Active? Young People and Health-enhancing Physical Activity — Evidence and Implications*. HEA, London

Health Education Board for Scotland (2000) *Indicators for Health Education In Scotland: Summary of findings from the 1998 Health Education Population Survey*. HEBS, Edinburgh

Health Media News (2001) *Fresh evidence for benefits of fruit*. http://www.health-secure.net (accessed June 2001)

Hunt K, Ford G, Mutrie N (2001) Is sport for all? Exercise and physical activity patterns in early and late middle age in the West of Scotland. *Health Educ* **101**(4): 151–8

Hussey J, GormleyJ, Bell C (2001) Physical activity in Dublin children aged 7–9 years. *Br J Sports Med* **35**: 268–73

Irving LM, Neumark-Sztainer D (2002) Integrating the prevention of eating disorders and obesity: feasible or futile? *Prev Med* **34**: 299–309

Jeffry S (2001) Nutrition: The role of the nurse in obesity management *JCN Online* **15**(3) http://www.jcn.co.uk (accessed March 2002)

Josefson D (2001) Obesity and inactivity fuel global cancer epidemic. *Br Med J* **322**: 945

Kant AK, Schatzkin A, Grawbard BI (2000) A prospective study of diet quality and mortality in women. *JAMA* **283**: 2109–15

Koikkalainen M, Mykkanen H, Julkunen J, Saarinen T, Lappalainen R (2002) Changes in eating and weight control habits after myocardial infarction. *Patient Educ Counselling* **26**:125–130

Koivusilta LK, Rimpela AH, Rimpela MK (1999) Health-related lifestyle in adolescence — origin of social class differences in health? *Health Educ Res* **14**(3): 339–55

Kuribayashi A, Roberts MC, Johnson RJ (2001) Actual nutritional information of products advertised to children and adults on Saturday. *Children's Health Care* **30**(4): 309–22

Lyubomirsky S, Casper RC, Sousa L (2001) What triggers abnormal eating in bulimic and non-bulimic women? *Psychol Women Q* **25**: 223–32

Manson JE *et al* (1999) A prospective study of walking as compared with vigorous exercise in the prevention of coronary heart disease in women. *N Engl J Med* **341**: 650–8

Mercer SW, Tessier S (2001) A qualitative study of general practitioners' and practice nurses' attitudes to obesity management in primary care. *Health Bulletin* **59**(4) http://www.schotland.gov.uk/health/cmobulletin/hb594-09asp (accessed January 2002)

Miilunpalo S, Nupponen R, Laitakari J, Marttila J, Paronen O (2000) Stages of change in two modes of health-enhancing physical activity: methodological aspects and promotional implications. *Health Educ Res* **15**(4): 435–48

Miles A, Rapoport L, Wardle J, Afupe T, Duman M (2001) Using the mass media to target obesity: an analysis of the characteristics and reported behaviour change of participants in the BBC's 'Fighting Fat, Fighting Fit' campaign. *Health Educ Res* **16**(3): 357–72

Mind Out for Mental Health http://www.mindout.net (accessed March 2002)

Narayan KM, Bowman BA, Engelgau ME (2001) Prevention of type 2 diabetes. *Br Med J* **323**: 63

Nauta H, Hospers H, Jansen A (2001) One-year follow-up effects of two obesity treatments on psychological well-being and weight. *Br J Health Psychol* **6**: 271–84

Ogden J, Bandura I, Cohen H, Farmer D, Hardie J, Minas H, Moore J, Qureshi S, Walter F, Whitehead MA (2001a) General practitioners' and patients' models of obesity: whose problem is it? *Patient Educ Counselling* **44**: 227–33

Ogden J, Baig S, Earnshaw G, Elkington H, Henderson E, Linsday J, Nandy S (2001b) What is health? Where GPs' and patients' worlds collide. *Patient Educ Counselling* **45**: 265–9

Parmenter K (2000) Changes in nutrition knowledge and dietary behaviour. *Health Educ* **102**(1): 23–9

Plonczynski DJ (2000) Measurement of motivation for exercise. *Health Educ Res* **15**(6): 695–705

Povey R, Conner M, Sparks P, James R, Shepherd R (2000) Application of the theory of planned behaviour to two dietary behaviours: roles of perceived control and self-efficacy. *Br J Health Psychol* **5**: 121–39

Romans MC (1997) Physical activity and exercise among women. *Women's Health Issues* **7**(1):

Rousseau ME (2001) Evidence-based practice in women's health: hormone therapy for women at menopause. *J Midwif Women's Health* **46**(3): 167–80

Rudolf MCJ, Sahota P, Barth JH, Walkjer J (2001) Increasing prevalence of obesity in primary school children: cohort study. *Br Med J* **322**: 1094–5

Sahota P, Rudolf MCJ, Dixey R, Hill AJ, Barth JH, Cade J (2001a) Randomised controlled trial of primary school based intervention to reduce risk factors for obesity. *Br Med J* **323**: 1–5

Sahota P, Rudolf MCJ, Dixey R, Hill A, Barth JH, Cade J (2001b) Evaluation of implementation and effect of primary school based intervention to reduce risk factors for obesity. *Br Med J* **323**: 1–4

Sparling PB, Owen N, Lambert EC, Haskell WL (2000) Promoting physical activity: the new imperative for public health. *Health Educ Res* **15**(3): 367–76

Tanne JH (1999) One diet fits all. *Br Med J* **318**: 1646

Telegraph (2001) *More obese adults in the UK.* http://www.telegraph.co.uk (accessed June 2001)

Teitz CC (2000) Fitness over Forty: Minimising risks in sports and exercise. *Women's Health in Primary Care* **3**(9): 629–39

Vuori I (1998) Does physical activity enhance health? *Patient Educ Counselling* **33**: 95–103

Wardle J (1995) Parental influences on children's diets. *Proceedings of the Nutrition Society* **54**: 747–58

Wardle J, Huon G (2000) An experimental investigation of the influence of health information on children's taste preferences. *Health Educ Res* **15**(1): 39–44

Weist J, Lyle RM (1997) Physical activity and exercise: a first step to health promotion and disease prevention in women of all ages. *Women's Health Issues* **7**(1): 10–16

Wood D, DeBacker G, Faergeman O, Graham I, Mancia G, Pyorala K (1998) Prevention of coronary heart disease in clinical practice: Recommendations of the second joint task force of European and other societies on coronary prevention. *Eur Heart J* **19**: 1434–1503

Woods MF, Mitchell ES (1997) Preventative Health Issues: The perimenopausal to mature years (45–64). In: Allen KM, Phillips JM, eds. *Women's Health: Across the lifespan.* Lippincott, Philadelphia: chapter 5

Woolf-May K, Kearney EM, Owen A, Jones DW, Davison RCR, Bird SR (1999) The efficacy of accumulated short bouts versus single daily bouts of brisk walking in improving aerobic fitness and blood lipid profiles. *Health Educ Res* **14**(6): 803–15

Wyn R, Solis B (2001) Women's health issues across the lifespan. *Women's Health Issues* **11**(3): 148–159

4

Maintaining a healthy liver

Introduction

Many people do not appreciate that the abuse of alcohol causes much more harm than illegal drugs like heroin and cannabis. It is a major tranquilliser, addictive and can cause physical illness and accidents. Physical illnesses attributed to alcohol abuse are gastritis, haematemesis, liver disease and some forms of cancer. Psychologically, alcohol can make people depressed and many of those who commit suicide also have alcohol problems (BBC News, 1999). Drinking in excess of four units per day for men and three units per day for women is sufficient to cause health problems (Twigg *et al*, 2000). This chapter focuses on the prevalence of excessive and abusive drinking in women and young people and the health consequences of abusing alcohol.

Health consequences of the abuse of alcohol

Common adverse effects of heavy alcohol consumption:

❖ Liver cirrhosis and liver cancer.

❖ Mouth, throat, gullet and possibly breast cancer.

❖ High blood pressure and related conditions such as heart and kidney disease, and stroke.

❖ Complications of pregnancy and infancy.

❖ Mental illness, suicide, epilepsy and damage to the nervous system.

❖ Accidents.

❖ Violence.

(Source: Department of Health, 1999)

Key facts about people and alcohol

❖ Not only are more children in Scotland drinking, they are drinking more.

❖ Four out of ten children aged fifteen had had a drink in the last week.

❖ Boys drink more than girls.

❖ Children who drink frequently are more likely to report drug use.

❖ Young people are the most likely age group to exceed weekly recommended limits.

❖ Two out of three young men and one out of two young women drank more than twice the recommended daily benchmarks on their heaviest drinking day.

❖ The commonest place of purchase of alcohol by children in Scotland (aged twelve to fifteen) was the off-licence, followed by shop or supermarket. One in five children aged twelve to fifteen are buying alcohol directly from a friend or relative.

❖ In 2000, there were 1,428 emergency admissions of young people aged ten to nineteen with a diagnosis of acute intoxication.

❖ People living in the most deprived areas were twice as likely to be admitted as a psychiatric inpatient with an alcohol-related diagnosis than those living in the least deprived areas.

❖ Alcohol-related death rates for women have doubled in the last decade.

❖ One in five road accident deaths in Scotland is due to drink driving.

❖ One in three adult pedestrian fatalities had alcohol levels over the legal limit for driving.

❖ Misuse of alcohol was a contributory factor in over 50% of deaths caused by fire in Scotland.

(Source: Statistics on alcohol in Scotland, 2002)

In the UK, 38% of men and 21% of women consume more alcohol than the recommended daily benchmarks and 26% of men and 15% of women exceed weekly recommendations (BHF, 2002). Only 10% of the population are teetotal and there are approximately 200,000 dependent drinkers in the UK. To place UK alcohol consumption in some context, it is reported that on average the UK consumption is less than that of France but more than the United States. In 1997, using litres per head, the figures for UK, France and USA are as follows: 7.5; 11.5; 6.6 (Scottish Executive, 2002).

There are approximately 33,000 premature deaths in England and Wales attributed to excessive alcohol consumption. Alcohol associated with 80% of suicides, 50% of murders, 80% of deaths from fire, 40% of road traffic accidents, 30% of fatal road traffic accidents and 15% of drowning. Alcohol contributes to one in three divorces, one in three cases of child abuse and 20–30% of all hospital admissions (Ashworth and Gerada, 1997).

The death figures related to alcohol abuse in Ireland are reported to be 150 people every year and a further 600 to 700 deaths attributed partly to alcohol misuse. In the document, *Investing for Health* (DHSSPS, 2002), it is reported that 82% of men and 72% of women consume alcohol and 25% of men and 14% of women drink in excess of the recommended limits. The proportion of teenagers who have tasted alcohol is stated to be 90% in the fifteen to sixteen-year-old age group. Furthermore, when asked if they had consumed alcohol in the last month, 70% of boys and 66% of girls, again in the fifteen to sixteen-year-old age group, admitted that they had (DHSSPS, 2002).

It is reported that one in four adults in the UK misuse alcohol. Men were more likely to have indulged in hazardous drinking (38%) compared with only 15% of women. The figures for Scotland demonstrate that the majority of adults drink alcohol with 74% of men and 53% women reporting having a drink in the last week. Scottish men and women are more likely to have drunk more than twice the recommended daily benchmarks than those in England.

The figures associated with hazardous drinking reveal 26% of women and 44% of men drinking double or more the recommended levels on their heaviest drinking days (Scottish Executive, 2002). When Scottish and English figures are compared, the gender differences are 24% males compared to 20% males in England, and 12% women compared to 8% women in England.

The British Heart Foundation (2002) states that 21% of women consume more alcohol than the recommended levels of between two and three units a day. There is evidence of age differences: 41% of women in the sixteen to twenty-four age group drink more than the recommended levels compared with 4% of women over sixty-five years of age.

A unit refers to the amount of alcohol found in a half pint of beer, lager or cider, a short of whisky or other spirits, a small glass of wine or sherry. A unit of alcohol equates to 8 grams by weight or 1cl (10mls) by volume of pure alcohol (DoH, 2001). Extra strong lagers and beers have double the units as ordinary ones. It should also be considered, that measures poured at home are usually larger than those served in pubs. Rather worryingly, a recent survey conducted in Scotland discovered that only 35% of men and 51% of women were aware of the correct recommended daily levels of alcohol (SE, 2002).

Again, there is a regional and gender difference with the highest rate of drinking over the recommended intake of alcohol manifesting in women in Scotland and the north-west of England and the lowest in London and the eastern region. The British Heart Foundation (2002) offer the example of 27% of women in Scotland consuming more than three times the recommended levels on the heaviest drinking day of the week compared to 16% of women in eastern England.

Women in professional occupations are three times as likely to drink over the recommended levels than women in unskilled occupations. Roxburgh (1998) attributes this to job demands and excessive time pressures. She reports that degrees of demands at work, amount of job control available on the job and how challenging and varied the work is all contribute to work-related stress which in turn may influence alcohol consumption. Women who have heavy drinking partners are at greater risk of becoming heavy drinkers themselves. Pregnant women who consume alcohol are placing their foetus at risk. The risks are less clearly identified with low and moderate consumption, but heavy alcohol consumption is associated with foetal alcohol syndrome and giving birth to a child with learning disabilities (Wyllie and Casswell, 1997).

Irish men and women are more likely to exceed recommended levels than those in the general population with 56% of Irish women reported to exceed the guidelines on the heaviest drinking day. Smith *et al* (2000) suggest that religion may have an influence on drinking alcohol in ethnic groups since, 'religious limits are placed on... drinking alcohol among Muslims... Sikh male levels of drinking reflect the absence of specific Sikh prohibition on alcohol' (p. 399).

Coleman and Hendry (1999) state that in present day society, alcohol consumption among teenagers is common. In England, 46% of young men and 35% of young women report having had an alcoholic drink at least once by the time they were fifteen years of age. The DoH (2001) in the preliminary results of *Drug use, smoking and drinking among young people in England in 2001*, reported that the prevalence of drinking alcohol in those aged eleven to fifteen years old rose from 21% in 1998 and 1999 to 24% in 2000 and 26% in 2001. They note that the increased prevalence was more noticeable among the thirteen to fifteen-year-olds as opposed to the eleven- to twelve-year-olds. Some 28% of boys and 25% of girls had drunk alcohol in the last week. The average consumption in 1990 was 5.3 units. In 2001, the average rate in boys was 10.6 units and 8.9 units in girls, giving an overall average of 9.8 units.

The majority of teenagers only drink alcohol a few times a year and mostly under parental supervision. It is seen as part of the socialisation into adulthood (Coleman and Hendry, 1999). However, there are teenagers who attempt to buy alcohol. Coleman and Hendry (1999) report that 25% of fifteen-year-old pupils stated that they had purchased alcohol from a supermarket or off-licence in the previous week and 10% had bought alcohol in a pub. Teenagers report that they drink alcohol to relax, increase their sociability and for the sensory and cognitive changes it produces (Coleman and Hendry, 1999). Kloep *et al* (2001) add boredom and 'nothing to do' and group pressure to this list. They continue by noting that young people perceive drinking alcohol as a skill to be learnt and that hangovers are an inevitable consequence of the learning process.

Alcohol is stated to be the most widely used drug among young people. Perry *et al* (2002) note that there is a strong correlation between alcohol consumption and many social and behavioural problems such as fighting, truancy, depression, self-harm and suicide. Alcohol consumption among women in the UK is rising. Teenage girls are among the heaviest drinkers in Europe (Plant and Haw, 2000). Between the years 1984 and 1998, the percentage of women in the age band sixteen to twenty-four who consumed alcohol rose from 15% to 25%. Plant and Haw (2000) report that in 1999, 78% of Scottish fifteen-year-old girls had been intoxicated and 56% reported that they had had five or more consecutive alcoholic drinks in the preceding month.

Plant and Haw (2000) report the findings of a four-year ethnographic study conducted by Barnes-Powell (1997). The study involved working class women in the age group twelve to twenty-one in central England. The researcher found that young women's developing drinking patterns were inextricably linked to their daily lives and their social position. These young women perceived drinking alcohol as being liberating, providing them with power, more confidence and improving their ability to express themselves. Alcohol was also seen as a mood-setter and disinhibitor.

Finally, being drunk provided time-out from the reality of life. Makela and Mustonen (2000) found that men report how drinking helped them to increase their social attractiveness by being funny and witty. Women reported that drinking helped them express their feelings and sort out their interpersonal problems.

Based on a Finnish adolescent health life style survey in 1999 of 2,385 participants, it was noted that drunkenness was more common in smokers than non-smokers. The researcher, Lintonen *et al* (2001) suggested the reason for this may be related either to individual vulnerability towards the formation of addictions or to the socialisation with substance using peers.

Lintonen *et al* (2001, p. 165) proposed a portrait of a potential heavy drinker as:

> *He/she is probably a smoker, living with a family with little parental control but ample spending money to hand out to the adolescent. He/she may be biologically more mature than his/her friends and has started dating.*

Plant and Haw (2000) remark that in the UK, older women tend to either have stopped drinking or were abstainers. Older drinkers view alcohol almost entirely as a positive act. Since alcohol has a greater effect on older women as a group, they experience more alcohol problems at lower levels of drinking, particularly accidents and falls. They also take longer to recover from bouts of heavy drinking.

The pattern of drinking in the UK involves heavy or binge drinking at the weekend but little during the week. This pattern of drinking is believed to result in greater harm and is associated with drunkenness and convictions for alcohol-related driving in addition to admissions to psychiatric units, alcohol-related injuries and premature deaths (Plant and Haw, 2000). Binge drinking can be defined as the consumption of five or more alcoholic drinks in a row on at least one occasion.

Norman *et al* (2000) describe binge drinking as consuming half of the recommended weekly level in one single session. Recent research from the United States suggests that the habit of binge drinking can cause rapid damage to brain cells (BBC News Online, 2002). The Joseph Rowntree Foundation conducted a recent survey involving 14,000 English secondary school-age children. Alarmingly, they found that binge drinking occurs in teenage children. It was reported that 25% of thirteen- to fourteen-year-olds and nearly 50% of fifteen- to sixteen-year-olds admitted to binge drinking at least once in the previous week (BBC News Online, 2002).

In Norman *et al*'s (2000) research involving 136 undergraduate students, they found that 46.3% reported binge drinking on at least one occasion per week. Of those, around 70% were males and 30% females. Males were reported to have a more positive attitude towards binge drinking, viewing it as a way of socialising with friends.

It was thought that the reason why women experience less alcohol-related harm than men was due to the fact that women tended to drink lower levels of alcohol. However, Plant and Haw (2000) report a recent study in which women experience lower levels of alcohol-related harm, regardless of the level of alcohol intake. Furthermore, Ely *et al* (1999) state that the probability of having drink-related problems increases with the level of consumption and is significantly greater for women. Ely *et al* (1999) suggest the physical factor of variation in the amount of body water as an explanation.

A high alcohol intake has a neuro-toxic effect. Up to 40,000 people are thought to die prematurely as a consequence of drinking alcohol to excess. Smoking and alcohol consumption increases the risk of oesophageal cancer forty-four times (Bennett and Murphy, 1997). Prolonged heavy alcohol consumption is a major cause of cirrhosis and a risk factor for hypertension and cancers (Health Education Board for Scotland [HEBS], 2000). The revised sensible limits of twenty-eight units for men and twenty-one units for women is being challenged by the British Medical Association who would prefer to remain with the previous limits of twenty-one and fourteen for men and women respectively (Bennett and Murphy, 1997). Plant and Haw (2000) report that many people do not understand the sensible drinking messages. They report a survey conducted in Scotland which demonstrated that while the majority of adults had heard of units, less than 33% could correctly identify how many units were in one pint of beer.

Women with severe alcohol problems often have multiple problems, including post-traumatic stress disorder and other psychiatric disorders. Plant and Haw (2000) state that it is essential that these problems are identified and addressed within any treatment regimen.

Despite the health problems cited above, it is suggested that a moderate intake of alcohol has a number of positive effects: antioxidant, lipo-protein and anti-thrombolytic effects which may be responsible for the reduced risk of stroke in those individuals who drink in moderation (Anon, 2001).

Alcohol is believed to be associated with a reduced risk of coronary heart disease but only if taken in moderation (one or two drinks per day). This is evidenced by the fact that rates for coronary heart disease are lower in France despite similar rates of animal fat consumption in both countries. Epidemiological evidence suggests that moderate consumption of red wine may offer cardio-protective benefit (Anon, 2001). If those levels are exceeded or people indulge in binge drinking, then the risk is greater. Boback *et al* (2000) report the findings of their study of beer drinkers. They found that the lowest risk of developing myocardial infarction was found in men who drank almost daily or who drank between four and nine litres of beer a week. However, in line with other studies, moderation was the key as they suggest that the protective effect of alcohol was lost in men who drank twice a day or more.

Ruitenberg *et al* (2002) report on their prospective population based study of 7,983 individuals over the age of fifty-five. They found that those who consumed up to three glasses of alcohol per day had a lower risk of dementia and vascular dementia than those who never drank alcohol.

Suggested web resources

http://www.alcoholics-anonymous.org.uk
http://www.show.scot.nhs.uk/nca The Nursing Council on Alcohol was launched in November 2000 and is dedicated to developing knowledge and awareness of alcohol-related problems
http://www.wrecked.co.uk Think about drink

References

Anon (2001) Exercise helps prevent cognitive decline. *Women's Health in Primary Care* **4**(11): 722

Ashworth M, Gerada (1997) ABC of mental health: Addiction and dependence – II: Alcohol. *Br Med J* **315**: 358–60

Barnes-Powell (1997) *Young Women and Alcohol: Issues of pleasure and power.* University of York, York

BBC News (1999) *Doctors declare war on male suicide 13th October.* http://news.bbc.co.uk/hi/english/health/newsid_25000/285131.stm (accessed April 2002)

BBC News Online (2002) *Binge drinking causes rapid brain damage.* http://www.bbc.co.uk (accessed October 2002)

Bennett P, Murphy S (1997) *Psychology and Health Promotion*. Open University Press, Aylesbury

British Heart Foundation (2002) *Coronary Heart Disease Statistics*. http://www.dphpc.ox.ac.uk/bhfthprg/stats/2000/2002/index.html (accessed February 2002)

Boback M, Skodova Z, Marmot M (2000) Effect of beer drinking on risk of myocardial infarction: population based case-control study. *Br Med J* **320**: 1378–9

Coleman LM, Hendry R (1999) Exploring young people's difficulties in talking about contraception: how can we encourage discussion between partners? *Health Educ Res* **14**(6): 741–50

Department of Health (1999) *Saving Lives. Our Healthier Nation*. DoH, London

Department of Health (2001) Drug use, smoking and drinking among young people in England 2001: Preliminary Results. http://www.doh.gov.uk/public/press15march02htm (accessed March 2002)

Department of Health, Social Services and Public Safety (2002) *Investing for Health*. http://www.dhsspsni.gov.uk/publications/2002/investforhealth.html (accessed March 2002)

Ely M, Hardy R, Longford NT, Wadsworth MEJ (1999) Gender differences in the relationship between alcohol consumption and drink problems are largely accounted for by body water. *Alcohol Alcoholism* **34**(6): 894–902

Health Education Board for Scotland (2000) *Indicators for Health Education In Scotland: Summary of findings from the 1998 Health Education Population Survey*. HEBS, Edinburgh

Kloep M, Hendry LB, Ingebrigtsen JE, Glendinning A, Espnes GA (2001) Young people in 'drinking' societies? Norwegian, Scottish and Swedish adolescents' perceptions of alcohol use. *Health Educ Res* **16**(3): 279–91

Lintonen TP, Konu AI, Rimpela M (2001) Identifying potential heavy drinkers in early adolescence. *Health Educ* **101**(4): 159–68

Makela K, Mustonen H (2001) Relationships of drinking behaviour, gender and age with reported negative and positive experiences related to drinking. *Addiction* **95**(5): 727–36

Norman P, Conner M, Bell R (2000) The theory of planned behaviour and exercise: evidence for the moderating role of past behaviour. *Br J Health Psychol* **5**: 249–61

Perry CL, Williams CL, Komro KA, Veblen-Mortenson S, Stigler MH, Munson KA, Farbakhsh K, Jones RM, Forster JL (2002) Project Northland: long-term outcomes of community action to reduce adolescent alcohol use. *Health Educ Res* **17**(1): 117–32

Plant M, Haw S (2000) *Women and Alcohol: report of an expert seminar*. Health Education Board and Alcohol and Health Research Centre, Edinburgh

Roxburgh S (1998) Gender differences in the effect of job stressors on alcohol consumption. *Addict Behav* **23**(1): 101–7

Ruitenberg A, van Swieten JC, Witteman CM, Mehta KM, van Duijn CM, Hofman A, Breteler MMB (2002) Alcohol consumption and risk of dementia: the Rotterdam Study. *Lancet* **359**: 281–6

Scottish Executive (2002) *Statistics on Alcohol in Scotland*. http://www.scotland.gov.uk/health (accessed February 2002)

Smith GD, Chaturvedi N, Harding S, Nazroo J, Williams R (2000) Ethnic inequalities in health: a review of UK epidemiological evidence. *Crit Public Health* **10**(4): 375–408

Twigg L, Moon G, Duncan C, Jones K (2000) Consumed with worry: 'unsafe' alcohol consumption and self-reported problem drinking in England. *Health Educ Res* **15**(5): 569–80

Wyllie A, Casswell S (1997) Gender focus of target groups for health promotion strategies in New Zealand. *Health Promotion Int* **12**(2): 141–9

5

Maintaining mental health

How society works at every level influences the way people feel about themselves. And how people feel influences how well society functions.

(Scottish Executive, 1999, p. 15)

Introduction

Of the many contexts in which gender is defined and enacted, a particularly important one is our relationship with others. Our earliest relationships in families weave our gender into our basic self-concepts. Later in life, we form friendships and romantic relationships in which we express our gendered identities. We participate in professional associations in which gender may affect how we act and how others perceive and treat us. Relationships and gender influence each other so that relationships define gender, and in turn, sculpts the character of relationships.

In Western cultures women are believed to be more emotionally expressive in general than are men. Specifically, they are expected to smile more as well as to show more sadness, fear, and guilt. In contrast, men are believed to show more overt emotional displays only in terms of physically aggressive anger. These gender stereotypes appear to be socialised into children's belief systems as early as three to five years.

(Hess *et al*, p. 610)

This chapter addresses the variety of factors which contribute to experiencing mental health problems and health promotion initiatives which can help to ameliorate distressing systems.

Definition of terminology

Public mental health involves exploring ways in which to create a mentally healthy society (DoH, 2001c). The Mental Health Promotion Project (DoH, 2001e) offers the following definitions of relevant terms:

Mental health: '... more than the absence of mental illness. There are many different definitions of mental well-being and these are influenced by individual experiences and expectations, as well as by cultural and religious beliefs. Mental health influences how we think and feel about ourselves and others and how we interpret events. It affects our capacity to learn, communicate, and to form and sustain relationships. It also influences our ability to cope with change, transition and life events — having a baby, going to prison, experiencing bereavement. Mental health may be central to all health and well-being, because how we think and feel has a strong impact on physical health' (p. 28). There is, for example, a link between psychosocial well-being and the development of coronary heart disease. Four areas are highlighted as being particularly involved: depression; social support; work-related stress and personality type. Working in jobs with a high level of stress and/or a lack of control increases the risk of developing coronary heart disease and dying prematurely. Poor social support can have a detrimental effect on health and recovering from illness (DoH, 1999).

Mental health promotion: 'involves any action to enhance the mental well-being of individuals, families, organisations or communities... (it is) essentially concerned with how individuals, families, organisations and communities think and feel, the factors which influence how we think and feel, individually and collectively, and the impact that this has on overall health and well-being' (p. 27). Effective mental health promotion depends on expertise, resources and partnerships across all sectors and disciplines (SE, 1999).

Mental health problems: '... are often defined in relation to specific diagnoses, for example, depression or schizophrenia. However, a mental health problem can refer to any problem that disrupts the way we think and feel, either temporarily, for example following a bereavement, or on a more severe and enduring basis' (p. 28). Depression and anxiety are one of the most common mental health problems which 5% of the population within the UK will suffer every year (Sherbourne *et al*, 2001). Keeley (2000) estimates that in any year, 25% of the population are at risk of experiencing a mental health problem.

Contributing factors to developing mental health problems

In the document, *Our Healthier Nation*, genetic, socio-economic, lifestyle and environmental factors, as well as access to services are cited as contributing to the development of mental health problems. The absence of clear career and life pathways for those who are unemployed is believed to be a reason why unemployed people have a tendency to be more emotionally unstable and, indeed, may lead them to doubt the value of their existence (Fergusson *et al*, 2001). From the Prison Reform Trust study, *Troubled Inside*, it was evident that nine out of ten young offenders have at least one mental health problem and over 50% of young male remand prisoners have a mental health disorder (Ananova, 2001).

Mental health promotion

The Department of Health (2001e) set up the mental health promotion project with the aim of improving the mental well-being of the general population of the UK, increasing social inclusion of people with mental health problems by tackling discrimination and finally, reducing the death rate from suicide by at least a fifth by 2010. To facilitate meeting the aim, a national service framework was developed which required all local services to develop their own local mental health promotion strategy by March 2002 (Stark *et al*, 2002). The National Service Framework devised a number of standards and two are particularly relevant here. Standard one relates to mental health promotion and standard seven relates to preventing suicide.

Some key facts

❖ Unemployed people have twice the risk of experiencing depression than those in employment.

❖ Children in the poorest households are at three times greater the risk of mental health problems than those in more affluent households.

❖ Half of all women and a quarter of all men will be affected by depression at some time in their lives.

❖ Individuals who have been abused or been victims of violence have higher rates of mental health problems.

❖ Between 25% and 50% of those individuals who sleep rough or in night shelters may have a serious mental health problem and up to 50% may additionally have alcohol dependence.

❖ People who have drug and/or alcohol problems usually have higher rates of other mental health problems.

❖ People with physical illnesses have higher rates of mental health problems.

❖ Every week 10% of the UK population aged sixteen to sixty-five report significant depressive symptoms, one in ten admit to suicidal thinking but fewer than two people in a million will kill themselves.

❖ Depressive disorders are common, but suicide remains rare.

(Source: DoH, 2001e; Davies, 2002)

The aim of standard one: Mental health promotion is to ensure health and social services promote mental health and reduce the discrimination and social exclusion associated with mental health problems... Health and social services should promote mental health for all, working with individuals and communities (and) combat discrimination against individuals and groups with mental health problems and promote their social inclusion (DoH, 2001e, p. 10). Mental health promotion is therefore most effective when it works at strengthening social networks and empowering individuals and local communities. The mental health promotion project document, *Making It Happen — A guide to delivering mental health promotion*, states that mental health promotion works at three levels:

1. Strengthening individuals to increase their emotional resilience through interventions to promote self-esteem and life and coping skills.
2. Strengthening communities, thereby increasing social inclusion and participation, improving neighbourhood environments, developing health and social services which support mental health, anti-bullying strategies at school, child care and self-help.
3. Reducing structural barriers to mental health by reducing discrimination and inequalities, promoting access to education, meaningful employment, housing, services and supporting those who are vulnerable.

In the document, *Making It Happen — A guide to delivering mental health promotion* (DoH, 2001e), both protective and risk factors are identified and presented in *Tables 5.1* and *5.2*.

Women have a greater risk than men for developing depression, anxiety, eating disorders and self-harm. The reported rates of depression and anxiety are higher in women than in men but the explanation remains unclear (Griffin *et al*, 2002). It is known that women's speech is based on notions of equality, supportiveness, expression of feelings, inclusivity, responsiveness and personal discourses. Women are more likely to confide about their private thoughts and problems to their same sex friends than men. The WHO (2000a) suggest that the fact that women bear the burden of responsibility associated with being wives, mothers and carers of others, coupled with the likelihood that they are in poorly paid employment may provide an answer.

According to the National Service Framework for Mental Health (1999), one in six people within the UK will experience some form of mental health problem in their lifetime, making mental illness as common as asthma. The *NHS Plan* (DoH, 2000) cites a figure of one in four. The most common types of problems are anxiety and depression. One in 250 people will have a psychiatric disorder such as schizophrenia or a bipolar disorder (manic-depression). The incidence of mental health problems including emotional, conduct and eating disorders in children and adolescents is one in five (Yamey, 1999).

Table 5.1: Protective factors potentially influencing the development of mental health problems and mental disorders in individuals (particularly children)

Individual factors	Family factors	School context	Life events and situations	Community and cultural factors
Easy temperament	Supportive caring parents	Sense of belonging	Involvement with significant other person (partner/mentor)	Sense of connectedness
Adequate nutrition	Family harmony	Positive school climate	Availability of opportunities at critical turning points or major life transitions	Attachment to and networks within the community
Attachment to family	Secure and stable family	Pro-social peer group	Economic security	Participation in church or other community group
Above-average intelligence	Small family size	Required responsibility and helpfulness	Good physical health	Strong cultural identity and ethnic pride
School achievement	More than two years between siblings	Opportunities for some success and recognition for achievement		Access to support services
Problem-solving skills	Responsibility within the family (for child or adult)	School norms against violence		Community/cultural norms against violence
Internal locus of control	Supportive relationship with other adult (for a child or adult)			
Social competence	Strong family norms and morality			
Social skills				
Good coping skills				
Optimism				
Moral beliefs				
Values				
Positive self-related cognitions				

Table 5.2: Risk factors potentially influencing the development of mental health problems and disorders in individuals (particularly children)

Individual factors	Family factors	School context	Life events and situations	Community and cultural factors
Prenatal brain damage	Having a teenage mother	Bullying	Physical, sexual and emotional abuse	Socio-economic disadvantage
Prematurity	Having a single parent	Peer rejection	School transitions	Social or cultural discrimination
Birth injury	Absence of father in childhood	Poor attachment to school	Divorce and family break up	Isolation
Low birth weight, birth complications	Large family size	Inadequate behaviour management	Death of family member	Neighbourhood violence and crime
Physical and intellectual disability	Antisocial role models (in childhood)	Deviant peer group	Physical illness/impairment	Population density and housing conditions
Poor health in infancy	Family violence and disharmony	School failure	Unemployment, homelessness	Lack of support service, including transport, shopping, recreational facilities
Insecure attachment in infant/child	Marital discord in parents		Incarceration	
Low intelligence	Poor supervision and monitoring of child		Poverty/economic insecurity	
Difficult temperament	Low parental involvement in child's activities		Job insecurity	
Chronic illness	Neglect in childhood		Unsatisfactory workplace relationships	
Poor social skills	Long-term parental unemployment		Workplace accident/injury	
Low self-esteem	Criminality in parent		Caring for someone with an illness/disability	
Alienation	Parental substance misuse		Living in nursing home or aged care hostel	
Impulsivity	Parental mental disorder		War or natural disaster	
	Harsh or inconsistent discipline style			
	Social isolation			
	Experiencing rejection			
	Lack of warmth and affection			

One way of measuring levels of depression, anxiety, sleep disturbance and happiness is to use the General Health Questionnaire (GHQ12) which has proven to be a valid and reliable tool. Gaining a score of four or more indicates a high level of psychological distress. Women tend to have a slightly higher score than men (18% compared to 13%) and the scores tend to be higher in both genders over seventy-five. Individuals with a low income tend to have a higher score indicating psychological distress than those with higher incomes. The BHF (2002) report that the Bangladeshis have the highest levels of psychological distress followed by Pakistanis. Some 30% of Bangladeshi women have high levels of psychological distress and black Caribbean women are also reported as having higher levels of psychological distress than women in the general population.

According to the report *Health in Scotland* (SE, 2001), mental health problems in children and adolescents are significantly associated with poverty and social exclusion. A survey performed by the Office of National Statistics demonstrated that 10% of children between the ages of five and twenty-five had some form of mental health problem. Five per cent had clinically significant conduct disorders, 4% had anxiety or depression and 1% were assessed as hyperactive. Boys were more affected than girls. Mental health promotion has a role in preventing mental health problems especially anxiety, depression, drug and alcohol dependence and suicide. Conduct disorder is a term used to describe a persistent and pervasive pattern of antisocial behaviour seen in childhood and adolescence. The prevalence is higher in boys (7%) than girls (3%), and occurs four times more often in individuals whose parent(s) are in unskilled occupations as opposed to professional ones. Typical behaviours expressed are disobedience, tantrums, destructiveness, lying and stealing. It is commonly associated with both social and educational disadvantage (Scott *et al*, 2001).

Anxiety and depression

Anxiety can be defined as, 'a mood state in which feelings of fear predominate and where the fear is out of proportion to any threat' and depression as, 'a negative mood state which involves a feeling of sadness' (NHS, 1999, p. 128–129).

It is estimated that one female in every fifteen and one male in every thirty will be affected by depression (DoH, 2001e). The incidence of depression is rising and one hypothesis put forward by @ease is the changes in society and culture and less emphasis on family life and social support. More than 20% of the population suffers from depression (@ease). Women have higher rates of depression and this is believed to be due to a disproportionate number of chronic stressors and negative life events coupled with fewer material and social resources (Griffin *et al*, 2002). Women who work full-time, especially those in managerial and professional roles, report more depressive symptoms than their counterparts who work part-time or are childless (Griffin *et al*, 2002). Even by controlling for marital status, number of children and number of dependants requiring care, Griffin *et al* (2002) found that women who had low control over their life had over twice the risk of depression than women who experienced high control. They concluded that low control at home, just like low control at work, affects the psychological morbidity of those involved.

Sherbourne *et al* (2001) report that anxiety in women often goes undetected and that women are twice as likely to suffer from depression than men. Elmore and Schneider (2001) and Hine (2001) support this. Sherbourne *et al* (2001) suggest that ethnic minorities and women with low socio-economic status are less likely to seek help for their depression or anxiety due to several factors including stigma, embarrassment and a belief that they can cope alone and/or that treatment will fail. Stigma seems to be one of the overriding factors, with loss of face being particularly acute in Asian Women (Barrett, 2001; Sherbourne *et al*, 2001). This is in contrast to findings from Albizu-Garcia *et al* (2001) who found that women are significantly more likely than men to seek help for an emotional or psychiatric disorder. They suggest that this may be due to socialisation processes in childhood in which girls become more perceptive of their feelings than boys. They also found that when men perceived their symptoms as causing significant morbidity, they sought help at a similar level to women. Mind Out for Mental Health (2002) report that 42% of people with a mental health problem do not inform their family members, 22% do not tell their partners, 74% do not mention it on application forms and 19% do not even tell their GP.

The Health and Safety Executive 1995 survey of self-reported work-related illnesses estimated that almost 300,000 people in the UK believe that they are suffering from work-related stress, anxiety or depression. Mind Out for Mental Health (2002) states that work-related stress ranks as the second highest occupational health problem after back problems, and that three in every ten employees will experience some kind of mental problem in any one year.

The key factors identified in the report were lack of control over work, monotony, pressure of work and exclusion from decision-making (NHS, 1999). Hemingway and Marmot (1999) assert that having control over one's work is more significant than either the pace or variety of tasks.

The BHF (2002) suggests that about 33% of women experience a high pace of work; are more likely to report a low level of variety at work than men and have less control over their work than men. Some 31% of women reported that they experienced low control compared to 19% of men. Women in social class V were three times more likely to report a lack of control over their work than those in social class 1.

Anxiety can manifest itself in the form of panic attacks where individuals experience tachycardia, feelings of shakiness, sickness, and dyspnoea. Panic attacks can be particularly disabling and cause individuals to avoid going out of their home. Some individuals become anxious and fearful about an object or a situation and may develop a phobia. Others can experience anxiety in the form of obsessive compulsive disorder where, in order to control their feelings, they habitually perform certain behaviours over and over, for example, washing their hands or checking locked doors (Mind out for Mental Health, 2002).

Depression is associated with significant personal and economic costs and reported to be the leading cause of disability in women world-wide (American Psychological Association [APA], 2002). Depression manifests by a variety of symptoms such as loss of interest and motivation, anxiety, difficulty concentrating, feeling worthless, insomnia, early morning wakening, and alteration in appetite (Mind out for Health, 2002). In the UK six million people suffer from depression and it is predicted that by 2020, depression will be the second leading cause of disease burden. Presently, depression costs the NHS some £8 billion each year. Depression is caused by an imbalance in certain chemicals in the brain, which affects its metabolism. Additionally, genetics and a family history play a role along with life events. To address the chemical imbalance, antidepressants are used (e.mentalhealth.com). Depression in older people is often unrecognised as the older generation have been socialised not to 'bother' their GP with anything unless it is a physical complaint (Royal College of Psychiatrists, 2002).

Depression is an important cause of morbidity in females. Reading and Reynolds (2001) estimate that between 10% and 30%

of women with young children are affected. They cite a variety of causes including poor relationship with their partner; poor social support and stresses such as unplanned pregnancies, pre-term births, still-births and ill health of child. In their study of 271 families with young children, Reading and Reynolds (2001) found a close relationship between poverty and the incidence of depression in mothers with young children. E-mental-health.com state that 15% of people who are diagnosed with depression commit suicide and they cite the figure of 70% of all suicides in the UK as occurring in people who have depression. Rates of depression in women occur in midlife (APA, 2002).

Unemployment is also associated with increased vulnerability to suicide and parasuicide (Ostamo *et al*, 2001). Ostamo *et al* (2001) suggest that the rates of suicide attempts in the unemployed is ten times higher than the employed, while Naidoo and Wills (2000) suggest a figure of twice as high in the unemployed compared with the employed. Mental illness is an important causal predictor to some suicides. Approximately 25% of those who attempt suicide have been in contact with mental health care services in the preceding year.

Young men are more likely to commit suicide than young women with the figures of fifteen men in every 100,000 to 2.5 women in every 100,000. Again, areas of high deprivation have higher rates of suicide than other areas (SE, 2001).

Suicide

The World Health Organization estimates that every year, about 1 million people commit suicide and they expect this figure to rise to 1.5 million by 2020 (Brown, 2001). While more women are likely to attempt suicide, more men are successful principally due to the choice of more violent and active methods (BBC News, 1999).

In Scotland, the suicide rate for men under forty living in the most deprived socio-economic groups, has been rising over the last two decades. Scotland has the worst rates in this respect from the rest of the UK.

The Suicide Prevention Strategy for Scotland has been developed to tackle this problem and involves a multi-agency approach (SE, 2001). The suicide rate in young men remains worryingly high compared with twenty years ago and this group remains most at risk (Yamey, 2000).

Some key facts

❖ Men are three times more likely to commit suicide than women.

❖ Suicide rates among women in Scotland have fallen slightly since the 1970s and are now three times lower than rates in men. However, the proportion of women who kill themselves every year in Scotland is twice that in England and Wales.

❖ Young men are at particular risk of suicide. Suicide attempts have increased by 170% since 1985.

❖ Suicide is the leading cause of death in men between the ages of fifteen and twenty-four.

❖ Suicide is the second most common cause of death in men under thirty-five. The first cause is death in road traffic accidents.

❖ Men in unskilled occupations are four times more likely to commit suicide than those in professional occupations.

❖ Certain occupational groups, including farmers, health-care professionals and vets, are at an increased risk which is attributed to easier access to the means by which to commit the act.

❖ More than one in ten individuals with severe mental illness commit suicide.

❖ Suicide rates in prisons are high.

❖ One per cent of patients who are seen in hospital due to incidents of self-harm, proceed to commit suicide during the following twelve months.

❖ Alcohol misuse is thought to be a major factor in the strikingly high rates of suicide found in some European countries in transition, for example, the Baltic and Russia.

(Sources: Brown, 2001; Appleby *et al*, 2001; Christie, 2001; DoH, 2001e; Mind out for Health, 2002; Stark *et al*, 2002)

The main causes of suicide attempts are due to inter-personal relationship problems, lack of finances, poor self-esteem, social support, and feelings of loneliness (Naidoo and Wills, 2000; Ostamo *et al*, 2001). According to a study by psychiatrists in Imperial College, London, the suicide rate in males between the ages of fifteen and nineteen have increased by more than 70%. They report a rise in hangings from a figure of fourteen in 1970 to fifty-four in 1998, suggesting that hanging is the most popular method of committing suicide (*The Times*, 2001). The following matrix illustrates the variety of differences in demography, rates and methods used to commit suicide in England and Wales, Northern Ireland and Scotland.

	England and Wales	Northern Ireland	Scotland
Annual suicide rate	10.0 per 100,000	9.9 per 100,000	17.3 per 100,000
Commonest methods in males	Overdose, hanging	Overdose, hanging, drowning	Overdose, hanging, drowning
Use of violent methods such as hanging, jumping from a height or in front of a moving vehicle	Men = 57% Women = 39%	Men = 5% Women = 52%	Men = 63% Women = 40%
Percentage single	38%	38%	35%
Percentage widowed	7%	6%	9%
Percentage divorced/ separated	26%	27%	27%
Percentage married	29%	29%	30%
Unemployed/long-term sickness	59%	60%	59%

(Source: Appleby *et al*, 2001)

Prevention strategies

Standard seven of the National Service Framework for Mental Health focuses on the prevention of suicide. The aim of the standard is, 'to ensure that health and social services play their full part in the achievement of the target in *Saving Lives: Our Healthier Nation* to reduce the suicide rates by at least one fifth by 2010'. The standard reads: 'local health and social care communities should prevent suicides by:

* promoting mental health for all, working with individuals and communities (standard one)
* delivering high quality primary mental health care (standard two)

- ensuring that anyone with a mental health problem can contact local services via the primary care team, a helpline or an A&E department (standard three)
- ensuring individuals with severe and enduring mental illness have a care plan which meets their specific needs, including access to services round the clock (standard four)
- providing safe hospital accommodation for individuals who need it (standard five)
- enabling individuals caring for someone with severe mental illness to receive the support which they need to continue to care (standard six).

And, in addition:

- support local prison staff in preventing suicides among prisoners
- ensure that staff are competent to assess the risk of suicide among individuals at greatest risk
- develop local systems for suicide audit to learn lessons and take any necessary action.

(DoH, 2001e)

The prevention of suicide has been a NHS priority since 1992, but until now there was no comprehensive strategy drawn up. Appleby *et al* (2001) in their document, *Safety first: Five-year report of the national Confidential Inquiry into Suicide and Homicide by People with Mental Illness* recommend that a broadly-based suicide prevention strategy is required for each country in the UK.

The European Union is considering targeting three specific groups in its campaign against suicides. The three groups are firstly those with mental health problems; secondly, those who misuse alcohol, solvents and drugs; and thirdly, those who have deliberately self-harmed as they have a high risk of suicide, estimated at 100 times greater than that of the general population (Watson, 2000).

One of the targets in *Our Healthier Nation* is to reduce the death rate from suicide by at least 17% by 2010, which equates to a reduction of 800 less deaths per year (Keeley, 2000). Car fumes are noted by Keeley (2000) as becoming increasingly used by young men in their suicide attempts and he suggested that this justifies the Government's policy initiative to reduce exhaust emissions. Fitting catalytic converters to reduce the carbon monoxide content in petrol powered cars is thought to be responsible for some of the fall in male suicides (Yamey, 2000).

Another policy initiative, which appears to have reduced the number of suicides, is making it harder to purchase large quantities of paracetamol and aspirin. The legislation, introduced in 1998, restricted pharmacists to selling a maximum of thirty-two tablets per sale (previously no restriction) and restricted other retail outlets to selling a maximum of sixteen tablets, where previously the limit had been twenty-four (Hawton *et al*, 2001). The rationale related to the belief that since self-poisoning was often a highly impulsive act, associated with a low suicide intent and a limited knowledge of the effects that such overdoses can have, that by limiting the availability, the number of overdoses would be reduced (Hawton *et al*, 2001).

An Oxford study reported by *The Telegraph* in 2001 found that deaths from paracetamol and aspirin poisoning had dropped by 20% and 50% respectively. They also found that liver transplants resulting from paracetamol overdoses had reduced by over 60%. Hawton *et al* (2001) conducted a prospective study to investigate the impact of the legislation on mortality from paracetamol or salicylates overdoses. They found that the number of deaths from self-poisoning with paracetamol alone and with salicylates alone reduced following legislation. They also found that there was a reduction in the number of liver transplants and admissions to liver units with hepatic paracetamol poisoning.

The number of deaths caused by sniffing volatile substances has gradually fallen over the past ten years in England and Wales. Barratt (2001) reports that the annual death rate in 1990 was 152 and this fell to seventy-three in 1999. Sniffing volatile substances is more common in boys than in girls. Barratt further reports that the number of deaths from sniffing was 258 in England and Wales between 1995 and 1999 compared with seventy-eight ecstasy-related deaths in the same time period. The commonly misused item in sniffing is butane from refill canisters for cigarette lighters. Although legislation was introduced in 1994 banning the sale of such refills to people less than eighteen years of age, they were responsible for 53% of deaths from sniffing in 1999 (Barratt, 2001).

The Department of Health has funded a pilot helpline in Manchester called CALM (campaign against living miserably) which offers a safety net for young men with mental health problems. The helpline is staffed by trained counsellors and aims to tackle the stigma attached to mental illness and increase the uptake of services available (NHS, 1999). The CALM helpline is open from 5.00 pm until 3.00 am on a freephone number (0800 585858). The calmzone.net, a Scottish helpline was launched in April 2002, at a cost of £1.2

million from the Scottish Executive, which aims to overcome the macho culture that leads to the bottling up of problems. Its target population is mainly men in the age group of fifteen to forty (*Daily Record*, 2002).

It is reported that 71% of people who are contemplating suicide would prefer to talk face-to-face with someone about their problems. Only 8% would choose a telephone helpline and a meagre 1% a website. The Samaritans have walk-in help centres where individuals can talk face-to-face with trained counsellors but, unfortunately, many people only associate the Samaritans with a telephone helpline (BBC News, 1999).

In 1998, the Royal College of Psychiatrists launched a five-year national campaign designed to reduce the stigma attached to mental illness in both the public and professional health arenas.

The campaign is called 'Changing Minds – every family in the land' and a series of booklets have been produced on a variety of topics such as anxiety, depression, schizophrenia, Alzheimer's disease, dementia, anorexia nervosa, bulimia, alcohol and drug misuse with a view to increasing understanding and reducing stigma (NHS, 1999).

Another active campaign against stigma and discrimination surrounding mental illness is Mind out for Mental Health who argue that labels are for things and not for people. In the *NHS Plan* (2001) it is noted that 55% of young people would not want anyone else to know if they had a mental health problem, and 47% of people with a mental health problem have experienced discrimination at work.

Improving public understanding plays an important role in reducing stigma and discrimination of those with mental health problems. There is a growing belief that individuals who have mental health problems should be supported within the community by integrated services (Mind Out for Mental Health). Mind Out for Mental Health states that discrimination is particularly powerful in areas of employment, housing and access to services. They point out that unemployment rates in those with long-term mental health problems are much higher than those who have an equivalent long-term physical disability and that this contributes to social exclusion. Only 13% are in employment compared to 33% in other long-term health problems. Mind out for Mental Health is a Department of Health funded national anti-discrimination campaign working closely with partners in the voluntary sector, the media, companies and youth and student organisations to combat the stigma and discrimination surrounding mental health. Their aim is to raise awareness, challenge people's assumptions and provide practical advice to help people make positive changes in their attitudes and behaviour.

As media coverage can have a profound effect, it is vital that they are involved in any campaign at awareness raising and initiatives to change attitudes. In 1997, a Health Education Authority report found that almost 50% of national press coverage during 1996 linked mental health problems with violence and criminality. The Press Complaints Commission's 'Code of practice' states that the press should avoid prejudicial or pejorative references to a person's race, colour, religion, sex or sexual orientation or to any physical or mental illness or disability. Mind Out for Mental Health (2002) assert that the latter is regularly flouted.

Mental health problems in children

Scott *et al* (2001) state that the commonest psychiatric disorder in children is conduct disorder, which has a prevalence rate of 7% in boys and 3% in girls. Children with conduct disorder typically exhibit behaviours such as tantrums, disobedience, fighting, destructiveness, lying and stealing. The disorder is most commonly associated with social and educational disadvantage and Scott *et al* (2001) note that it is four times more common in families with unskilled occupations compared to professional ones.

Children with conduct disorder are likely to have reading difficulties and leave school either without educational qualifications or are excluded for their anti-social behaviour. In 40% of eight-year-olds, this anti-social behaviour persists leading to convictions for theft, assault and vandalism (Scott *et al*, 2001).

Experimenting with illicit drugs

The Health Development Agency (HDA) (1997) reports that experimenting with illicit drugs appears widespread in secondary schools with children commencing around the age of thirteen. In 2001, 6% of eleven-year-olds had used drugs in the last year and 39% of fifteen-year-olds had done so (DoH, 2001f). HDA (1997) note that drug education does not occur until fourteen to sixteen. In 2001, 12% of pupils reported that they had used drugs in the previous month and 20% reported drug use in the previous year. The

Government strategy for tackling drug misuse has a target to reduce the proportion of young people under twenty-five misusing Class A drugs by 25% by 2005, and 50% by 2008 (DoH, 2001f). In the document *Drug use, smoking and drinking among young people in England in 2001*, the following information is provided about Class A drugs. Class A drugs are considered to cause the most harm. The most common drug to be used in 2001 was cannabis.

Drug	Mode of use	Classification
Amphetamines	inject	A
Ecstasy	oral	A
Cocaine	sniff or inject	A
Crack	inject or smoke	A
Heroin	smoke, sniff or inject	A
LSD	oral	A
Magic mushrooms	oral	A
Methadone	oral	A
Amphetamines	sniff or oral	B
Cannabis	smoke or oral	B
Tranquillisers	oral or inject	B/C (depends on drug)
Anabolic steroids	oral or inject	C

Motives given by children for using drugs include:

- curiosity
- drug use seen as fun and exciting
- peer pressure and the need to conform
- belief that drugs will help them cope with problems (HDA, 1997).

Boys *et al* (2001) report results from the most recent British Crime Survey in which reasons for illicit drug use were identified as:

- to relax (96.7%)
- to become intoxicated (96.4%)
- to keep awake at night while socialising (95.7%)
- to enhance an activity (88.5%)
- to alleviate a depressed mood (86.8%).

Boys *et al* (2001) also report that approximately 50% of young people between the ages of sixteen and twenty-four have used an illicit drug at least once. The most prevalent illicit drug used is cannabis. The percentage of drug use in respect of age groups can be seen below.

Drug	Sixteen to nineteen age group	Twenty to twenty-four age group
Cannabis	40%	47%
Amphetamine sulphate	18%	24%
LSD	10%	13%
Ecstasy	8%	12%
Cocaine	3%	9%

The Government's (1998) ten-year strategy on drug misuse, *Tackling Drugs to Build a Better Britain*, identifies young people as a critical priority group for prevention and treatment interventions (Boys *et al*, 2001).

The HDA (1997) summary outlined interventions which should be adopted. These are listed below:

- target specific needs of, and particular groups of young people
- target a range of settings, audiences and substances both within and outside school environments
- students aged between eleven and thirteen should be included in target groups
- programmes should be intensive, lasting up to about fifteen hours and include regular booster sessions
- programmes should emphasise that drug use is neither as prevalent nor as acceptable as young people believe
- programmes should have a mixture of elements, including social influences and skills training
- finally, messages must be credible and not delivered by uniformed police officers.

The drug misuse figures for adolescents in Scotland are provided in the document *Health in Scotland* (SE, 2001). In the twelve to fifteen age group, 17%–18% have taken drugs at some time, 14%–15% have taken drugs in the last year, and 10% have taken drugs in the last month. There appears to be an increase in use in fifteen-year-olds as opposed to twelve-year-olds as it is reported that only 1% of twelve-year-olds had used drugs in the last month, compared to 22% of fifteen-year-olds. The report states that boys were more likely to have been offered drugs than girls.

There is a strong age gradient in drug misuse. Younger age groups are much more likely to misuse drugs. The highest prevalence is in the sixteen to twenty-four age group and there is a substantial decrease in prevalence towards the fifty-five to seventy-four-year-old age group (HEBS, 2000).

Forty per cent of men and 36% of women agreed that they did not know enough about the risks associated with taking drugs. It is interesting to note that the group expressing greatest need for information was the one most likely to have parenting responsibility for teenagers (HEBS, 2000).

There are a number of key elements in tackling the problem of drug misuse. HEBS (2000) outlines three principal aims:

- raising awareness and understanding about drugs and drug-related issues, focusing on young people and parents
- promoting attitudes and behaviours which encourage abstinence from illicit drugs
- encouraging alternatives to illicit drug use.

Promoting mental health

For children with conduct behaviour disorder, several initiatives have been implemented. 'Surestart' programmes target children between nought and three years of age with a one-stop shop service for parents. 'On Track' programmes aim to prevent anti-social behaviour in four- to twelve-year-olds, thereby preventing crime later on. Health action zones aim to reduce exclusion in school, drug use and early pregnancy. Scott *et al* (2001) advocate strongly for a well co-ordinated multi-agency approach to ensure effectiveness.

The Strategy for Adolescent Mental Health Services, is the first all-Wales strategy which aims to improve the range and quality of services for children and young people with emotional and behavioural problems by promoting a partnership approach across health, social care, education and the voluntary sectors (WHO, 1997).

There are several initiatives used in promoting mental health. MIND, the mental health charity, promotes mental health through education and produces a series of readable and jargon-free booklets aimed at carers and users. Occupational health personnel in workplaces can promote mental health in their workforce (Keeley, 2000). The Department of Health Priorities Framework for 2002/2003 (2001c) include:

❖ By 2004 all people with a serious mental illness will be able to access a Crisis Resolution Team twenty-four hours a day, seven days a week.

❖ By 2004 all young people who develop a serious mental illness will be in receipt of Early Intervention Services. All people who regularly disengage from services leading to frequent relapse and occasionally, offending behaviour will be in receipt of Assertive Outreach services by December 2003.

❖ Increased capacity by 2004 through: 500 more community mental health staff, 700 more staff to support carers, 300 staff working in prisons, and 1000 newly trained primary care mental health workers.

Suggested web resources

http://www.depressionalliance.org/
http://www.phs.ki.se Health promotion research Internet network with links WHO Collaborating Centre for suicide research and prevention
http://www.mentalhealth.org.uk
http://www.mind.org.uk
http://www.rcpsych.ac.uk/public/help/welcome.htm Help is at hand
http://www.samaritans.org.uk/
http://www.trashed.co.uk
http://www.who.int/whr/2001 World Health Report 2001: mental health: new understanding, new hope

References

@ease http://www.at-ease.nsf.org.uk (accessed April 2002)
Albizu-Garcia CE, Alegria M, Freeman D, Vera M (2001) Gender and health services use for a mental health problem. *Soc Sci Med* **53**: 865–78
American Psychological Association (2002) Summit on Women and Depression: Proceedings and Recommendations. APA, Washington DC. http://www.apa.org/pi/wpo/women&depression.pdf (accessed April 2002)

Appleby L, Shaw J, Sherratt J, Amos T, Robinson J, McDonnell R (2001) *Safety First: Five Year Report of the National Confidential Inquiry into Suicide and Homicide by People with Mental Illness.* NICE and University of Manchester http://www.doh.gov.uk/mentalhealth/safetyfirst (accessed April 2002)

Barratt H (2001) Number of deaths from volatile substance misuse is falling. *Br Med J* **323**: 252

BBC News (1999) *Doctors declare war on male suicide 13th October.* http://news.bbc.co.uk/english/health/newsid_285000/285131.stm (accessed October 2002)

British Heart Foundation (2002) *Coronary Heart Disease Statistics.* http://www.dphpc.ox.uk/bhfthprg/stats/2000/2002/keyfacts/index.html (accessed February 2002)

Boys A, Marsden J, Strang J (2001) Understanding reasons for drug use amongst young people: a functional perspective. *Health Educ Res* **16**(4): 457–69

Brown P (2001) Choosing to die — a growing epidemic among the young. *Bull World Health Organ* **79**(12): 1175–7

Christie B (2001) Suicide rate in young men in Scotland is twice that in England and Wales. *Br Med J* **323**: 888

Daily Record (2002) *New helpline to cut suicide toll.* 11 March. http://www.health-news.co.uk (accessed March 2002)

Davies S, Naik PC, Lee AS (2001) Depression, suicide and the national service framework. *Br Med J* **322**: 1500–1

Department of Health (1999) *Saving Lives: Our Healthier Nation.* DoH, London

Department of Health (2000) *The NHS Plan: A plan for investment, a plan for reform.* CM4818, HMSO, London

Department of Health (2001a) *The Annual Report of the Chief Medical Officer of the Department of Health 2001: On the State of the Public Health.* DoH, London

Department of Health (2001c) *Priorities and Planning Framework 2002/2003.* DoH, London http://www.doh.gov.uk/planning2002-2003/index.htm (accessed January 2002)

Department of Health (2001e) Mental Health Promotion Project: Making it Happen: A guide to delivering mental health promotion. DoH, London. http://www.doh.gov.uk/mentalhealthpromotion/index.htm (accessed March 2002)

Department of Health (2001f) *Drug use, smoking and drinking among young people in England 2001: Preliminary Results.* http://www.doh.gov.uk/public/press15march02.htm (accessed March 2002)

Elmore KO, Schneider RK (2001) Anxiety disorders in Women. *Women's Health in Primary Care* **4**(11): 691–8

Fergusson DM, Horwood J, Woodward LJ (2001) Unemployment and psychosocial adjustment in young adults: causation or selection? *Soc Sci Med* **53**: 305–20

Griffin JM, Fuhrer R, Stansfeld SA, Marmot M (2002) The importance of low control at work and home on depression and anxiety: do these effects vary by gender and social class? *Soc Sci Med* **54**: 783–98

Hawton K, Townsend E, Deeks J, Appleby L, Gunnell D, Bennewith O, Cooper J (2001) Effects of legislation restricting pack sizes of paracetamol and salicylate on self poisoning in the United Kingdom: before and after study. *Br Med J* **322**: 1–7

Health and Safety Executive 1995

Health Development Agency (1997) *Health promotion in young people for the prevention of substance misuse. Health promotion effectiveness reviews Summary Bulletin* 5 http://www.hda-online.org.uk/html/research/effectivenessreviews/erereview5.html (accessed January 2002)

Health Education Agency (1998) *Young and Active? Young People and Health-enhancing Physical Activity — Evidence and Implications*. HEA, London

Health Education Board for Scotland (2000) *Indicators for Health Education In Scotland: Summary of findings from the 1998 Health Education Population Survey*. HEBS, Edinburgh

Hemingway H, Marmot M (1999) Psychological factors in the aetiology and prognosis of coronary heart disease: a systematic review of prospective cohort studies. *Br Med J* **318**: 1460–7

Hess U, Senecal S, Kirouac G, Herrera P, Philipott P, Kleck RE (2000) Emotional expressivity in men and women: stereotypes and self-perceptions. *Cognition and Emotion* **14**(5): 609–42

Hine D (2001) National perspective: United Kingdom. *Women's Health* **11**(4): 293–9

Keeley P (2000) Mental Health Promotion. In: Kerr J , ed. *Community Health Promotion: Challenges for Practice*. Baillière Tindall, London: chapter 9

Mind Out for Mental Health http://mindout.net (accessed March 2002)

Naidoo J, Wills J (2000) Health Promotion: Foundations for Practice. 2nd edn. Baillière Tindall, London

National Health Service (1999) *National Service Framework for Mental Health: modern standards and service models*. http://www.doh.gov.uk/nsf/mentalhealth.html (accessed March 2002)

Ostamo A, Lahelma E, Lonnqvist J (2001) Transitions of employment status among suicide attempters during a severe economic recession. *Soc Sci Med* **52**: 1741–50

Reading R, Reynolds S (2001) Debt, social disadvantage and maternal depression. *Soc Sci Med* **53**(4): 441–53

Royal College of Psychiatrists (2002) *Depression in the Elderly*. http://www.rcpsych.ac.uk (accessed April 2002)

Scott S, Knapp M, Henderson J, Maughan B (2001) Financial cost of social exclusion: follow up study of antisocial children into adulthood. *Br Med J* **323**: 1–5

Scottish Executive (1999) *Public Mental Health Project*. Scottish Development Centre for Mental Health Services, Edinburgh

Scottish Executive (2001) *Health in Scotland*. http://show.scot.nhg.uk/publications (accessed February 2002)

Sherbourne CD, Dwight-Johnson M, Klap R (2001) Psychological distress, unmet need, and barriers to mental health care for women. *Women's Health* **11**(3): 231–43

Stark C, Mathewson F, O'Neill N, Oates K, Hay A (2002) Suicide in the Highlands of Scotland. *Health Bull* **60**(1) http://www.scotland.gov.uk/health/cmobulletin (accessed February 2002)

Telegraph (2001a) *Suicide rate drops following painkiller sales law*. Telegraph, 14 December. http://www.dailytelegraph.co.uk (accessed May 2001).

Times (2001) *Suicide rate up*. http:www.thetimes.co.uk (accessed September 2001)

Watson R (2000) EU aims to reduce suicides. *Br Med J* **321**: 852

World Health Organization (1997) *Strategy for Adolescent Mental Health Services*.WHO, Geneva

World Health Organization (2000a) *Women and Mental Health*. Fact Sheet No. 248. WHO, Geneva

Yamey G (1999) Mental health services are failing children and adolescents. *Br Med J* **319**: 872

Yamey G (2000) Suicide rate is decreasing in England and Wales. *Br Med J* **320**: 75

6

Healthy ageing

Introduction

This chapter focuses on the natural changes occurring in women as they grow older. This includes coverage of the peri-menopause, the menopause and the associated health issues.

Peri-menopause and menopause

The transition into the menopause is called the peri-menopause and it lasts a few years before and up to one year after the permanent cessation of menses. It is the peri-menopause that is associated with a reduction in circulating oestrogen and progesterone levels which in turn cause the range of symptoms experienced by women (Li *et al*, 2000).

The average age at which menopause occurs is fifty-one years, therefore women can expect to live for about a third of their lives in a hormonally deficient state. Women who smoke and/or are exposed to toxic chemicals, including those used in cancer chemotherapy, often reach the menopause earlier (Warren and Kulak, 1999).

There are a number of authors who challenge what they believe is the medicalisation of the menopause (Lee, 1998; Backett-Milburn *et al*, 2000; Klima, 2001). Lee (1998) asserts that since the menopause is a normal and healthy stage in a woman's life, it should be viewed as a symptom and not a disease to be treated. Klima (2001, p. 287) believes that since the menopause is labelled as a deficiency state, which requires hormone replacement therapy, it is seen as a disease to be managed rather than a natural process:

> *If women's health care is viewed through a deficiency lens, then it's likely that important aspects of the health of women may be overlooked in favour of the replacement approach. Models of deficiency tend to ignore the important role of the external environment, diet and activity level as important factors in health maintenance.*

Finally, MacLaren and Woods (2001) state that white women are more likely than black women to view medical intervention as appropriate for menopause.

The physical effects which women experience in the time leading to (perimenopausal) and during the menopause are due to the lower levels of circulating oestrogen. Low levels of oestrogen affect lipid metabolism which brings the risk of developing coronary heart disease to the same level as men (Lee, 1998). A lower level of circulating oestrogen also affects the reabsorption of calcium from bone leading to the development of osteoporosis.

Probably the most well known physical effect is hot flushes which 75% of perimenopausal women experience. Hot flushes (or hot flashes as they are known in North America) occur most frequently in the first two years of the menopause. They occur mostly at night causing sleep disturbance, which in turn can lead to fatigue, and depression.

Hot flushes also occur in warm environments, after the ingestion of caffeine or alcohol and during periods of stress (Warren and Kulak, 1999). Other physical effects of the menopause are atrophy of the genito-urinary tract and osteoporosis. The atrophy of the genito-urinary tract is due to a reduction in the circulating oestrogen level. The vagina, vulva, urethra and the trigone of the bladder all contain large numbers of oestrogen receptors so when the circulating oestrogen levels fall during the menopause all these areas atrophy.

The effects of the atrophy in turn cause a reduction in secretions, loss of elasticity and a reduction in the efficiency of muscles. These in turn cause dryness of the vagina, which can make sexual intercourse uncomfortable, or painful (dyspareunia) and increases the risk of vaginal and urinary tract infections. The loss of muscle efficiency can cause incontinence (Warren and Kulak, 1999).

Osteoporosis

As noted above, osteoporosis is the result of lower levels of oestrogen and its concomitant effect on calcium reabsorption. As the calcium levels in the bone reduce, the bone structure is weakened to a point where the bone can fracture easily. Osteoporosis is sometimes called the silent thief as bone mass is lost with no symptoms being felt until such time as a fracture occurs. Bone is constantly being created and broken down and during the time of peak bone mass development more is created than lost. By the mid-thirties peak bone mass will have been achieved and thereafter there is a slow reduction.

Key facts

❖ About three million people in the UK have osteoporosis (Schifrin, 2001).

❖ Bone loss begins earlier and proceeds more rapidly in females than in males, with an accelerated phase in the menopause (Ilich *et al*, 1996).

❖ World-wide, women have a 30–40% lifetime risk of osteoporosis compared to 13% in men (International Council of Nurses [ICN], 2001).

❖ Ten per cent of women over sixty years of age world-wide are affected by osteoporosis (ICN, 2001).

❖ A fifty-year-old white woman has a 15% risk of developing osteoporosis and by the age of eighty-five, 33% of white women will have suffered a fractured hip (Warren and Kulak, 1999).

❖ Osteoporosis is responsible for 200,000 fractures every year in the UK, costing the NHS £1.6 billion (Backett-Milburn *et al*, 2000; ICN, 2001).

❖ Every three minutes someone in the UK suffers a fracture as a result of osteoporosis and hip fractures account for more than 20% of orthopaedic bed occupancy (Schifrin, 2001).

❖ More women die a year as a result of osteoporotic fractures than from cancer of the breast and ovaries combined (ICN, 2001).

❖ Most common areas for osteoporotic fractures are the spine, hip, pelvis, upper arm and wrist (ICN, 2002).

❖ Osteoporotic wrist fractures occur in women more than men with a ratio of 5:1; crush fractures of spine have a ratio of 10 women to 1 man and fractures of the hip are twice as likely in women as they are in men (Ilich *et al*, 1996).

However, at the menopause where the oestrogen levels drop, there is acceleration in bone loss. By the menopause, many women will have lost about 30% of their bone mass. In the first five to ten years following the menopause, it is estimated that women may lose between 4% and 5% of bone per year (Warren and Kulak, 1999). It is important to note that the better the peak bone mass, the less vulnerable the individual will be to osteoporosis (Ilich *et al*, 1996; Weist and Lyle, 1997). To maintain healthy bone, an adequate calcium intake is required.

It is imperative that women are aware of the need to maintain an adequate intake of calcium in the years when they are developing their peak bone mass and, indeed, into later life. As Illich *et al* (1996, p. 202) state:

> *It is likely that variations in calcium nutrition early in life may account for as much as 5–10% difference in peak bone mass. Such a difference, although small, probably contributes to more than 50% of the difference in the hip fracture rates in later life.*

Risk factors in developing osteoporosis

There are a number of risk factors associated with developing osteoporosis. These are:

- being female, although men are vulnerable as well
- being fifty years old or older
- post-menopausal
- low life-time levels of oestrogen
- ovaries removed or menopause before the age of forty
- insufficient calcium intake
- limited exposure to sunlight or insufficient vitamin D intake
- limited physical activity, particularly weight bearing exercise
- family history of osteoporosis
- being thin or having a small frame
- being white or Asian
- tobacco use
- excessive caffeine intake
- excess alcohol intake.

(Source: Osborn *et al*, 1999; Backett-Milburn *et al*, 2000)

Preventing osteoporosis

Since osteoporosis cannot be cured, prevention is particularly important. It can be prevented by adopting a number of lifestyle changes, such as eating a well-balanced diet rich in vitamin D and calcium (between 1,000 and 1,300 mgs of calcium per day for females is suggested by Locke and Warren, 2000); not smoking, refraining from excessive alcohol and caffeine intake; and exercising, particularly resistance training and impact exercise prior to age thirty to encourage high levels of peak bone mass. Backett-Milburn *et al* (2000) also add the prevention of falls as being important, especially in the elderly. More than 300,000 individuals aged sixty-five or over attend A&E departments each year in England and Wales as a result of accidents at home, the majority of which are falls.

Between 5% and 10% result in fractures which are a major cause of morbidity and can lead to a reduction in the older person's independence (Evans, 2000). Evans suggests that an improvement in body posture through Tai Chi classes at day centres may help prevent falls. While, Backett-Milburn *et al* (2000) suggest that wearing polypropylene external hip protectors afford the frail elderly a degree of protection from hip fractures.

Hormone replacement therapy (HRT)

According to Warren and Kulak (1999) and Backett-Milburn *et al* (2000), in the USA, up to 30% of women take HRT for hot flashes and gain relief from symptoms. Schifrin (2001) states that 21.7% of English, 20.4% of Scottish, and 21.3% of Welsh women use HRT. HRT prevents bone loss by reducing the activity of osteoclasts and can reduce fracture rates by as much as 65% (Warren and Kulak, 1999). HRT also helps to reduce the risk of coronary heart disease in post-menopausal women by improving lipid levels (Lee, 1998). It is suggested that HRT lowers the risk of coronary heart disease by between 40–50% (Rousseau, 2001). However, it increases the risk of developing deep vein thrombosis and/or a pulmonary embolism by two to four times (Rousseau, 2001). On the other hand, a study by Margolis *et al* (2002) demonstrated that women over sixty-five years of age using HRT were about 30–40% less likely to develop venous leg ulcers than their counterparts who did not use HRT.

Lee (1998) states that at least six years of HRT is required to achieve a maximum benefit with regard to bone integrity and points out that after discontinuation of HRT rapid bone loss occurs. The Osteoporosis Society in Canada recommended at least ten years of HRT before the maximum protection is attained (Coo *et al*, 2001).

It is suggested by Lee (1998) that HRT may not be necessary if women undertake weight-bearing exercises and have an adequate calcium intake in the years before and after the menopause. There are other benefits to taking HRT. Recent research has revealed that HRT may help to prevent colon cancer, Alzheimer's disease and macular degeneration (Mahajan *et al*, 2001).

In order to make an informed decision one needs to have the available evidence in a form that one understands. Coo *et al* (2001) cite a Canadian study where a high proportion of women were aware that HRT may reduce the risk of osteoporosis but only a small proportion were aware that it could reduce the risk of coronary heart disease. Warren and Kulak (1999) point out a rather worrying figure of only one woman in every forty being aware of the increased risk of developing coronary heart disease following the menopause. Coo *et al* (2001) found that only about 60% of women were aware that HRT might increase the risk of developing breast cancer. A number of researchers (Barnard and Inkeles, 1999; Osborn *et al*, 1999; Villablanca, 2001) point out that although the risk is well documented it is thought to be small compared to the risk of coronary heart disease. Cobb (1998) states that statistically there is no doubt that a woman is more likely to die from coronary heart disease than breast cancer, and provides the figure as being about nineteen to one.

When they investigated where women gained their information about the effects of the menopause, it was from magazines and the media rather than from health professionals. Backett-Milburn *et al* (2000) found that unless women knew of someone with osteoporosis or had a family history of osteoporosis, they tended to be dis-interested in it as a health issue, which is very disappointing since prevention is so important to one's bone health in the longer term.

Healthy ageing

The UK is an ageing society. Since the 1930s the number of people aged sixty-five or over has more than doubled and one fifth of the population is over sixty years of age (DoH, 2001d). The Health Development Agency (1998) note that 18% of the UK population is sixty-five or older and the prediction is for this to rise to 23% by 2030. This represents a rise from 11 million to 14 million. By 2020 the population of Japan will be the oldest in the world with 31% being over sixty, followed by Italy, Greece and Switzerland (ICN, 2002).

Older people with better health habits live healthier for longer (McMurdo, 2000). The ICN (2002) defines good health and successful ageing in terms of, 'ability to function autonomously within a given social setting. If socially and intellectually active, the older person may be considered healthy even in the presence of chronic disease.' The best preparation for a healthy old age is advocated as a healthy middle age (SE, 2001).

Bryant *et al* (2001) attribute healthy ageing to: family, social contacts, physical health, mobility/ability, material circumstances, activities and happiness, youthfulness and home environment. They also note the importance of cultural expectations, environment, motivation and education as being contributory to healthy ageing.

Older people are most likely to define health as the ability to do things for themselves.

Staying healthy is not simply warding off illness. Rather, it is maintaining the ability to function in a community

(Arcury *et al*, 2001, p. 1553)

In a grounded theory study of twenty-two older people, Bryant *et al* (2001) found that being healthy, to these older people, meant going out and doing something meaningful. The concept had four components: having something worthwhile to do; the balance between abilities and challenges; appropriate external resources; and personal attitudinal characteristics. The latter was described as having a positive attitude as opposed to a 'poor me' one.

The ageing population has increased vulnerability to ill health due to a reduction in income, social isolation and age-related health problems. The leading causes of death in individuals sixty-five years of age and older, are coronary heart disease, cancer and stroke (Rice, 2000). Alzheimer's disease is the eighth leading cause of death. In the UK there are 325,000 individuals suffering from Alzheimer's disease (Schifrin, 2001). Older women have higher rates of Alzheimer's disease, osteoporosis and diabetes than older men (Lee, 1998).

Rice (2000) states that arthritis is the leading chronic condition with three out of five women suffering from it. The next leading cause is hypertension, followed by coronary heart disease. Clancy and Bierman (2000) state that half of women aged sixty-five or over report having two chronic conditions, while one in four report having three or more. They also report that there is a higher prevalence of chronic illness, co-morbidity, functional limitations and disability in older women in lower socio-economic groups. Arthritis is the leading cause of physical disability in the UK and its impact causes pain, fatigue, stiffness, inflammation which in turn leads to a reduction in physical functioning, impacts on work and social roles, which can lead to anxiety and depression, social withdrawal and social isolation (Barlow *et al*, 2001).

The *National Service Framework for Older People* is the first ever comprehensive strategy which aims to ensure fair, high quality, integrated health and social care services for older people. It is a ten-year programme of action linking services to support independence, promote good health, specialise services for key conditions and culture change so that all older people and their carers are always treated with respect, dignity and fairness (DoH, 2001d, p.1). In the framework, the Secretary of State for Health, Alan Milburn, refers to existing services, including free NHS sight tests for those sixty and over, an extension of breast screening availability for women aged seventy years and free influenza immunisation for everyone aged sixty-five and over.

The NHS Research and Development Strategic Review on ageing and age associated disease and disability (1999) predicts that if the prevalence of disability in later life continues at the current level, by the year 2013, there will be more than two million people in the UK who will require daily personal help. However, lessons can be learnt from the USA, where they have increased their emphasis on primary prevention of disabling diseases by the adoption of healthy lifestyles and preventative health care. The NHS Research and Development Strategic Review (1999) believes that this is worthwhile adopting in the UK since it appears to be making a difference in the USA.

The main health problems in older women are stroke, depression, hip fractures, osteoarthritis, coronary heart disease and urinary incontinence. Approximately 90% of all deaths in women due to coronary heart disease occur after the menopause (Lane *et al*, 1996). Women suffer more than men from depression and anxiety. Evans and Steptoe (2000) estimate that one in twenty women over retirement age experience depression.

The National Service Framework for Older People sets out standards for the care of older people across health and social services and the standards apply in whatever environment the older person is in. The standards specifically address conditions, which are particularly significant for older people (and not covered by other national service frameworks such as the one for coronary heart disease). The first standard relates to 'rooting' out age discrimination. The aim of this standard is to, 'ensure that older people are never unfairly discriminated against in accessing NHS or social care services as a result of their age.' The standard reads:

NHS services will be provided, regardless of age, on the basis of clinical need alone. Social care services will not use age in their eligibility criteria or policies, to restrict access to available services.

The rationale for this standard primarily focuses on the assertion that decisions about treatment and care should be made on the basis of each individual's health needs and ability to benefit, not their age.

The framework states that older people from black and minority ethnic groups can be particularly disadvantaged and the milestones set for health and social services are designed to address this.

Standard two of the framework is entitled person-centred care. It aims to:

... ensure that older people are treated as individuals and they receive appropriate and timely packages of care which meet their needs as individuals, regardless of health and social services boundaries... [and the standard reads] NHS and social care services treat older people as individuals and enable them to make choices about their own care. This is achieved through the single assessment process, integrated commissioning arrangements and integrated provision of services, including community equipment and continence services.

(p. 8)

The rationale for this standard is that with effective assessment of individual need and prompt provision of care, the older person's ability to function independently will be more likely to be preserved, rather than a premature admission to hospital or residential care.

Standard three on intermediate care reads:

Older people will have access to a new range of intermediate care services at home or in designated care settings, to promote their independence by providing enhanced services from the NHS and councils to prevent unnecessary hospital admission and effective rehabilitation services to enable early discharge from hospital and to prevent premature or unnecessary admission to long-term residential care.

(p. 10)

The rationale for this standard is the requirement for a new range of acute and rehabilitation services to bridge the gap between acute and primary and community care.

All older people who need hospital care should receive it. However, too many older people are admitted to hospital for the want of community based services that would better meet their needs. Consequently, they are running unnecessary risks of disruption to their social networks, disorientation and hospital acquired infections.

(p. 10)

The fourth standard on general hospital care reads:

Older people's care in hospital is delivered through appropriate specialist care and by hospital staff who have the right set of skills to meet their needs.

(p. 13)

This standard emphasises the need for the older person to be assessed, at an early stage, by a consultant in old age medicine or rehabilitation, so that treatment and management decisions can be made for them as an individual person who has specific needs relating to their ageing process.

Standard five relates to strokes. A stroke has a major impact on both the individual and their family. Nearly 20,000 people living in Scotland have been disabled by a stroke and 80% of these occurred when the individual was over sixty-five years of age. Stroke is now the main cause of neurological disability in the Scottish population (SE, 2001). Every year in England and Wales about 110,000 people have their first stroke and 30,000 people go on to have further strokes. Stroke is the single biggest cause of major disability. As with other diseases, some population groups are at greater risk than others. Not surprisingly, those in lower socio-economic groups are at greater risk than those in more affluent groups. African-Caribbean and South Asian communities are also at greater risk of developing a stroke. Stroke tends to be associated with older age groups but it can occur in younger people. For example, each year 10,000 people less than fifty-five years of age and 1,000 under the age of thirty experience a stroke. The fifth standard in the framework states that:

The NHS will take action to prevent strokes, working in partnership with other agencies where appropriate. People thought to have had a stroke have access to diagnostic services, are treated appropriately by specialist stroke services, and subsequently, with their carers, participate in a multidisciplinary programme of secondary prevention and rehabilitation.

(p.15)

The key aspect here is the hospital-based stroke unit, as there is strong evidence to suggest that people treated in such units are more likely to survive and have a much better prognosis that those who are admitted to non-specialist units (DoH, 2001d).

Standard six of the framework relates to falls. It reads:

The NHS working in partnership with councils, takes action to prevent falls and reduce resultant fractures or other injuries in their population of older people. Older people who have fallen receive effective treatment and, with their carers receive advice on prevention through a specialised falls service.

(p. 17)

Falls and their related injuries in older people are a cause of major health problems world-wide. It is estimated that 30% of people over the age of sixty-five will fall at least once a year and about half of these individuals will fall recurrently. Older people who fall are likely to sustain a fracture. About 90% of such fractures involve the hip (Khan *et al*, 2001). Every year in England, over 400,000 people attend A&E departments following an accident and up to 14,000 people a year die in the UK as a result of an osteoporotic hip fracture.

There are a number of risk factors associated with falls in older people. These are general physical functioning, gait, balance, sensory impairments, medical conditions and psychological, behavioural, and social factors (Khan *et al*, 2001). Part of the ageing process is the loss of muscle mass and hence muscle strength. McMurdo (2000) states that by the age of eighty about half of the muscle mass has gone.

Khan *et al* (2001) advise that physical training involving strength, balance and improved transfer will help to prevent falls. In addition, teaching people how to fall so as to minimise the risk of falling on their greater trochanter will reduce the likelihood of hip fracture. The introduction of specialised hip protector underwear can be of benefit in the prevention of hip fractures in the frail elderly.

In the 1994 General Household Survey, a gender difference to

Healthy ageing

functional abilities in the older population became evident. One fifth of men over eighty-five were unable to go out and walk down the street, while half of the women over eighty-five were unable to do so. Under 10% of men over eighty-five were unable to go up and down stairs, while 29% of women over eighty-five were unable to do so. The survey also identified a linear class gradient. Men who had previously been in semi or unskilled occupations prior to retirement were twice as likely to report their health as less than good, compared to their counterparts who had retired from non-manual occupations. The same held true for women (Arber and Ginn, 1998). Regular physical activity in old age can rejuvenate people (McMurdo, 2000).

McMurdo (2000) emphasises the importance of physical activity in the elderly, as a small loss of fitness following a period of illness can render an older person immobile and dependent. Even in extreme old age, lost fitness can be gained with regular physical activity and carers who insist on performing daily household duties for older people may in fact be doing them a disservice as this may be their only form of physical activity (McMurdo, 2000). *Investing for Health* (DHSSPS, 2002) reports that in Ireland, 28% of elderly people cannot participate in their chosen activities due to transport difficulties, particularly in rural areas.

Regular physical activity contributes to healthy ageing (Koltyn, 2001). Being physically active affords a number of positive benefits, particularly in the ageing population. It reduces biological changes associated with ageing, can control or improve chronic diseases, increases mobility and function and enhances rehabilitation from acute and chronic illnesses (Koltyn, 2001). Two studies (one from the USA and one Dutch) report that by maintaining exercise by walking regularly and exercising daily, the older age group are more likely to retain cognitive ability than those who do not exercise (International Herald Tribune, 2001; Reuters, 2001). Rather worryingly, the researchers noted that healthcare professionals tended to dissuade their ageing client group from exercising. Simey and Skelton (2001) suggest that four out of every ten people over the age of fifty are totally inactive. They state that even for the frailest individual, no exercise is a greater risk than being active and cite the Minister for Public Health as saying, 'exercise is the best buy in public health'. There are a number of initiatives which report that low intensity exercise programmes for the older members of society produces discernible health benefits even for the most severely disabled (McLaughlin, 2001; Parsons, 2001).

Standard seven of the framework is associated with mental

135

health in older people.

> *Older people who have mental health problems have*
> *access to integrated mental health services, provided by*
> *the NHS and councils to ensure effective diagnosis,*
> *treatment and support, for them and for their carers*

(p. 19)

The rationale for this standard refers to the fact that mental health problems of older people often remain under-detected as many live alone and symptoms of depression can be difficult to detect. 'Mental and physical problems can also interact in older people making their overall assessment and management more difficult' (p. 19).

The final standard of the framework relates to the promotion of health and active life in older age. The standard's aim is to extend the healthy life expectancy of older people.

> *The health and well-being of older people is promoted*
> *through a co-ordinated programme of actions led by the*
> *NHS with support from councils.*

(p. 21)

This standard relates to discussions in this chapter suggesting that:

> *There is a growing body of evidence to suggest that the*
> *modification of risk factors for disease even late in life can*
> *have health benefits for the individual; longer life, increased*
> *or maintained levels of functional ability, disease prevention*
> *and an improved sense of well-being. Integrated strategies*
> *for older people aimed at promoting good health and quality*
> *of life, and to prevent or delay frailty and disability can*
> *have significant benefits for the individual and society.*

(p. 21)

Promoting health in the older population can be achieved by visiting older people in their homes. Elkan (2001) reports that by offering health promotion and preventative care, death rates and admission to long-term institutional care are significantly reduced.

Suggested web resources

http://www.disability.gov.uk
http://disabilitynet.co.uk
http:www.abilitynet.co.uk
http://www.ageconcern.org.uk
http://weable.com

References

Arber S, Ginn J (1998) Health and Illness in Later Life. In: Field D, Taylor S, eds. *Sociological Perspectives on Health, Illness and Health Care*. Blackwell, Oxford: chapter 8

Arcury TA, Quandt SA, Bell RA (2001) Staying healthy: the salience and meaning of health maintenance behaviours among rural older adults in North Carolina. *Soc Sci Med* **53**:1541–56

Backett-Milburn K, Parry O, Mauthner N (2000) 'I'll worry about that when it comes along': Osteoporosis, a meaningful issue for women at mid-life? *Health Educ Res* **15**(2): 153–62

Barlow JH, Williams B, Wright CC (2001) Patient education for people with arthritis in rural communities: the UK experience. *Patient Education Counselling* **44**: 205–14

Barnard RJ, Inkeles SB (1999) Effects of an intensive diet and exercise program on lipids in postmenopausal women. *Women's Health* **9**(3): 155–61

Bryant LL, Corbett KK, Kutner JS (2001) In their own words: a model of health ageing. *Soc Sci Med* **53**(7): 927–41

Clancy CM, Bierman AS (2000) Quality and outcomes of care for older women with chronic disease. *Women's Health Issues* **10**(4): 178–91

Cobb JO (1998) Reassuring the women facing menopause: strategies and resources. *Patient Education Counselling* **33**: 281–8

Coo H, O'Connor KS, Hunter D (2001) Women's knowledge of hormone therapy. *Patient Education Counselling* **45**: 295–301

Department of Health (1997) *NHS R&D Strategy Review Ageing and Age-associated Disease and Disability: Report of the Topic Working Group*. DoH, London

Department of Health (2001d) *National Service Framework for Older People*. DoH, London. http://www.doh.gov.uk.nsf/olderpeople.htm (accessed March 2002)

Department of Health, Social Services and Public Safety (2002) *Investing for Health*. http://www.dhsspsni.gov.uk/publications/ (accessed March 2002)

Elkan R, Kendrick D, Dewey M, Hewitt M, Robinson J, Blair M, Williams D, Brummell K, Egger M (2001) Effectiveness of home-based support for older people: systematic review and meta-analysis. *Br Med J* **323**(7315): 719–25

Evans O, Steptoe A (2002) The contribution of gender-role orientation, work factors and home stressors to psychological well-being and sickness absence in male- and female-dominated occupational groups. *Soc Sci Med* **54**: 481–92

International Congress of Nurses (2001) ICN co-sponsors osteoporosis tour. ICN. *International Nursing Review* **48**: 201

International Congress of Nurses (2002) *ICN on Healthy Ageing: A public health and nursing challenge*. http://www.icn.ch/matters_aging.htm (accessed March 2002)

Ilich JZ, Badenhop NE, Matkovic V (1996) Primary prevention of osteoporosis: Pediatric approach to disease of the elderly. *Women's Health Issues* 6(4): 194–203

International Herald Tribune (2001) *Walking keeps older women alert*. http://www.iht.com (accessed May 2001)

Khan KM, Liu-Ambrose T, Donaldson MG, McKay HA (2001) Physical activity to prevent falls in older people: time to intervene in high risk groups using falls as an outcome. *Br J Sports Med* 35: 144–5

Klima CS (2001) Women's health care: A new paradigm for the 21st century. *J Midwif Women's Health* 46(5): 285–91

Koltyn KF (2001) The association between physical activity and quality of life in older women. *Women's Health Issues* 11(6): 471–80

Lane MJ, Macera CA, Croft JB, Meyer PA (1996) Preventive health practices and perceived health status among women over 50. *Women's Health Issues* 6(5): 279–85

Lee C (1998) *Women's Health: Psychological and Social Perspectives*. Sage, London

Li S, Holm K, Gulanick M, Lanuza D (2000) Perimenopause and the quality of life. *Clin Nurs Res* 9(1): 6–23

Locke RJ, Warren MP (2000) Good food for your bones. *Women's Health in Primary Care* 3(4): 297

MacLaren A, Woods NF (2001) Midlife women making hormone therapy decisions. *Women's Health Issues* 11(3): 216–30

Mahajan ST, Pinto AB, Williams DB (2001) The additional benefits of hormone replacement therapy. *Primary Care Update for OB/GYNS* 8(6): 260–3

Margolis DJ, Knauss J, Bilker W (2002) Hormone replacement therapy and prevention of pressure ulcers and venous leg ulcers. *Lancet* 359: 675–7

McLaughlin A (2001) Training showed noticeable improvement in elderly women. *Br Med J* 322: 798

McMurdo MET (2000) A healthy old age: realistic or futile goal? *Br Med J* 321: 1149–50

Osborn BH, Couchman GM, Siegler IC, Bastian LA (1999) Osteoporosis risk factors: Association with use of hormone replacement therapy and with worry about osteoporosis. *Women's Health Issues* 9(6): 278–85

Parsons M (2001) Exercise programmes benefit even those who are most severely disabled. *Br Med J* 322: 797

Reuters (2001) *Exercise may halt mental decline in the elderly*. http://www.reutershealth.com (accessed May 2001)

Rice DP (2000) Older women's health and access to care. *Women's Health Issues* 10(2): 42–6

Rousseau ME (2001) Evidence-based practice in women's health: hormone therapy for women at menopause. *J Midwif Women's Health* 46(3): 167–80

Schifrin E (2001) An overview of women's health issues in the United States and United Kingdom. *Women's Health Issues* 11(4): 261–81

Scottish Executive (2001) *Health in Scotland*. http://www.show.scot.nhs.uk/publications (accessed February 2002)

Simey P, Skelton D (2001) A healthy old age:realistic or futile goal? *Br Med J* 322: 796

Villablanca AC (2001) HRT and cardiovascular risk in women: Where do we stand? *Women's Health in Primary Care* 4(2): 121–9

Warren MP, Kulak J (1999) Benefits and drawbacks of hormone replacement therapy. *Women's Health in Primary Care* 2(1): 21–33

Weist J, Lyle RM (1997) Physical activity and exercise: a first step to health promotion and disease prevention in women of all ages. *Women's Health Issues* 7(1): 10–16

7
Maintaining sexual health

Introduction

Sexual health can be defined as, 'an essential component of general health and includes the avoidance of unintended pregnancies and sexually transmitted infections' (Nicoll *et al*, 1999, p. 1321). The DoH (2001g, p. 5) strategy states that:

> *Sexual health is an important part of physical and mental health. It is a key part of our identity as human beings together with the fundamental human rights to privacy, a family life and living free from discrimination. Essential elements of good sexual health are equitable relationships and sexual fulfilment with access to information and services to avoid the risk of unintended pregnancy, illness or disease.*

This chapter will discuss a variety of factors and diseases that affect the sexual health of women.

Sexual health

> *Sexual ill health affects all age groups and sections of society but harms disproportionately vulnerable groups such as young people, minority ethnic groups, and those affected by poverty and social exclusion.*
>
> (Kinghorn, 2001, p. 243)

The consequences of poor sexual health can be serious and have a long lasting impact on people's lives (DoH, 2001g). The DoH (2001g) 'National Strategy for Sexual Health and HIV' is the first in the UK to modernise sexual health and HIV services and aims at improving England's sexual health. The strategy is three-pronged with the development of primary care and user-friendly outreach centres to interlink and supplement existing specialist genito-urinary medicine services; the introduction of chlamydia screening and the extension of HIV testing to all antenatal and sexually transmitted infection clinic attendees. One-stop shops for the provision of comprehensive sexual health advice, contraception and testing for sexually transmitted infections will also be piloted (DoH, 2001g).

The consequences of poor sexual health

* Pelvic inflammatory disease, which can cause ectopic pregnancies and infertility.
* HIV.
* Cervical and other genital cancers.
* Hepatitis, chronic liver disease and liver cancer.
* Recurrent genital herpes.
* Bacterial vaginosis and premature delivery.
* Unintended pregnancies and abortions.
* Psychological consequences of sexual coercion and abuse.
* Poor educational, social and economic opportunities for teenage mothers.

(Source: DoH, 2001g)

Preventing poor sexual health requires people to be informed about ways that they can protect themselves. According to the DoH (2001g), education relating to maintaining sexual health is often uncoordinated and poorly targeted and the strategy serves as a vehicle to improve this. There are five areas within the strategy which reflect the Ottawa Charter for Health Promotion (1986):

1. Building healthy public policy that promotes sexual health at local and national levels and addresses inequalities.
2. Creating environments that are supportive of sexual health.
3. Developing personal and social skills regarding sex, sexuality and sexual health.
4. Ensuring that all services, which promote sexual health, build upon the evidence base and develop professionals' skills, knowledge and positive attitudes through education and training.
5. Strengthening community action in setting priorities, making decisions, planning strategies and implementing them to achieve better sexual health.

In July 1997, the Ottawa Charter was reviewed and the Jakarta Declaration was adopted with the aim of leading health promotion into the twenty-first century. The Jakarta Declaration identifies five priorities:

1. Promote social responsibility for health.
2. Increase investments for health development.
3. Expand partnerships for health promotion.
4. Increase community capacity and empower the individual.
5. Secure an infrastructure for health promotion (WHO, 1998a).

Sexual health information will be targeted, within the strategy, for specific groups as they are deemed to be more vulnerable, at higher risk or have particular access requirements. The specific groups include: young people, especially those in or leaving care; black and minority ethnic groups; gay and bisexual men; injecting drug mis-users; adults and children with HIV and other people affected by HIV; sex workers; and people in prisons and youth offending establishments (DoH, 2001g). The strategy outlines the action and targets of the Government, commissioners, service providers and health professionals (see overleaf).

Cancers

Cancer is caused when normal cell growth processes become abnormal. The reasons for the normal processes to alter and cause cancer are not fully understood but the causes are known to be complex (DoH, 1999). Naismith (1999, p. 2) states that:

> *The development of cancer is a multi-step process, a concept derived from animal experiments: initiation, promotion and progression. Substances capable of initiation are termed 'mutagens'. Promoters enhance the yield of tumours after exposure to the initiator, whereas progression is a complex process involved in the development of malignant groups of cells that have the capacity to disseminate and invade other tissues.*

In the UK, one in three people will be diagnosed with cancer at some time in their lives and one in four people will die of the disease.

'The Government will:

❖ Develop a new safer sex information campaign for the general population.

❖ Ensure national helplines on HIV and safer sex are more responsive to people's information needs.

❖ Use the work commissioned from the Health Development Agency to provide an evidence base for local HIV/STI prevention.

❖ Exploit the wide range of media available for providing information on sexual health.

❖ Set a target to reduce the number of newly acquired HIV infections.

❖ Develop, with London health authorities and others, a strategic framework for HIV prevention for African communities.

Commissioners, service providers and health professionals should:

• Focus sexual health promotion and HIV prevention on identified local need, set targets in line with national priorities and monitor progress as appropriate to local population

• Support all staff to develop their skills through work-based and other dedicated education and training programmes, in line with national priorities

• Ensure prevention is integral to service delivery

• Co-ordinate local information campaigns with national information campaigns and ensure they meet good practice benchmarks

• Work towards achieving a target to reduce the number of newly acquired HIV infections.'

(Source: DoH, 2001g, p. 21)

Despite the fact that the NHS spends around £1.5 billion every year on cancer care (Cancer Working Group, 1999), caccer survival rates in the UK generally lag behind those of Europe and the USA. Sikora (1999, p. 461) proposes some reasons why UK cancer survival rates are poorer than our comparable European neighbours. He proposes that it may be due to a delay in diagnosis, a delay in commencing treatment and/or the quality of cancer care and its integration. He states that:

If Britain could achieve the survival rates of the best country in Europe for each cancer, over 25,000 lives a year would be saved. Even if it could just reach the European average, nearly 10,000 lives would be saved.

There is also an inequality in survival, with better rates noted in those living in affluent areas as opposed to those living in more deprived areas (DoH, 1999). The Cancer Working Group (1999) also notes the effect of deprivation on survival rates (*Table 7.1*). They give the following examples:

Table 7.1: Examples of the effect of deprivation on survival rates

Site of cancer	Affluent area, five-year survival rate	Deprived area, five-year survival rate
Breast	71%	63%
Rectum	41%	35%
Hodgkin's disease	79%	72%

An explanation for the differing survival rates could be postulated to be due to poor general health, poor access or poor delivery of effective cancer treatment but as yet there is no empirical evidence to substantiate these hypotheses (Cancer Working Group, 1999).

Naismith (1999) provides information about the most common cancers in the UK expressed as a percentage of total cancers (*Table 7.2*).

Table 7.2: Percentage of common cancers in the UK

Site	Men	Women
Breast	0%	23%
Lung	22%	10%
Colorectal	12%	12%
Prostate	11%	0%
Stomach	6%	4%
Ovary	0%	4%
Cervix	0%	3%
Oesophagus	3%	3%

The DoH (1999) set a target of reducing the death rate from cancer in people under seventy-five years of age by at least 20% by 2010 which would mean saving some 100,000 lives. The most common killers are lung, breast, colorectal and prostate cancers which together amount to 62,000 deaths every year in the UK (DoH, 1999). The risk of developing cancer appears to be rising with nearly 200,000 new cases every year, however, the death rate from cancer appears to be falling. The latter is attributed to a better understanding of the mechanisms involved in its cause and prevention as well as improved screening and treatment (DoH, 1999). The DoH (1999) document expands upon this aspect by disclosing that the survival rate for a childhood cancer, acute lymphoblastic leukaemia rose from 10% thirty years ago to its current rate of over 70%. Other examples provided are the survival rate for Hodgkin's disease which nearly doubled from 30% to 55%, and that for cancer of the colon from 30% to 40%.

However, the increasing ageing population within the UK means that there will potentially be more cancer cases in the future. The Cancer Working Group (1999) projected the UK male and female cancer deaths based on the 1992 rates and produced the following statistics (*Table 7.3*).

Table 7.3: Projected UK male and female cancer deaths

	Year		
	1995	2002	2020
Lung cancer mortality	38,500	40,500	52,500
Breast cancer mortality	15,500	16,500	19,000
Bowel cancer mortality	20,000	21,000	27,000

It is estimated that 80% of cancers could actually be prevented (HEBS, 2001). The 'Health in Scotland' (2001) document contains five simple messages in relation to the prevention of cancer:

- do not smoke
- drink alcohol only in moderation
- eat more fruit and vegetables
- take regular exercise
- avoid over-exposure to sunlight.

These preventative factors are associated with the risk factors. Smoking tobacco, for example, causes most lung cancers and is implicated in many other types of cancer. In total, it is estimated that smoking causes about one third of all deaths attributed to cancer. Alcohol consumption increases the risk of cancer of the oral cavity, pharynx, larynx, oesophagus, breast and liver. It is generally believed that moderate alcohol (up to two drinks per day) will not appreciably increase the risk (Bandolier, 2002a).

According to the DoH (1999), low levels of consumption of fruit and vegetables are linked with an increased risk of colorectal and gastric cancer. Naismith (1999) explains the preventative qualities in fruit and vegetables as being the nutrients that they contain known as antioxidants, vitamins C, E and B-Carotene and Selenium. These antioxidants protect against free radicals that are generated in response to infections and smoking which in turn damage DNA and induce cancer development (Naismith, 1999). Kono (2001) however cautions this by suggesting that fruit and vegetables may have a protective effect against colorectal cancer but as yet there is no clear evidence.

Batty and Thune (2000) report that men and women who engage in physical activity have less than half the risk of developing cancer compared to their sedentary counterparts. It is proposed that physical activity reduces the risk of colon cancer because it reduces the transit time within the bowel and the contact time of the colon mucosa to faecal carcinogens (Batty and Thune, 2000). There is evidence that participating in regular exercise will reduce the incidence of coronary heart disease by a third, strokes by a quarter, non-insulin dependent diabetes by a quarter and hip fractures by a half (DHSSPS, 2002).

Avoiding over-exposure to sunlight is advocated in order to prevent skin cancer. The DoH (1999) states that being sunburnt as a child may result in an increased risk of skin cancer in adulthood. Ness *et al* (1999) report the findings from a survey conducted in 1995 which found that about 40% of individuals aged between sixteen and twenty-four reported being sunburnt in the proceeding year. In the UK, there are about 2000 cases of skin cancer per annum. The DoH (1999) report that users of sunbeds have between one and a half and two and a half times the risk of developing skin cancer. Women are reported to be more likely to contract melanoma skin cancer than men, but men are more likely to die from it (DoH, 1999).

Ness *et al* (1999) strongly argue that the messages regarding exposure to sunlight should be measured as while over-exposure is harmful, a lack of exposure can also have negative effects. They cite a Scottish study where 40% of individuals between the ages of twenty and thirty-five perceived having a sun tan made them feel healthy.

Ness *et al* (1999) continue by stating that exposure to the sun can be a relaxing and enjoyable experience; and can enhance the subjective feeling of well-being. They mention seasonal affective disorder (SAD), which causes depression, as being attributed to reduced exposure to ultraviolet light. Finally, they also mention the well-documented evidence of an increase in suicidal behaviour, which occurs in early spring, and suggest that one of the factors may be related to patterns of day length and sun exposure.

Obviously, to be aware of health promotion messages one has to understand them, and it is for this reason that the NHS cancer screening programmes have developed Braille versions and audio format of their leaflets for the blind and those who find reading difficult. Their leaflets have also been translated into five languages: Gujarati, Punjabi, Urdu, Bengali and Cantonese. A further twelve languages are to be available by the summer of 2002 in the form of downloadable pdf files from the cancer screening programmes website. These are Hindi, Somali, Polish, Turkish, Greek, Ukrainian, Arabic, Italian, Spanish, Vietnamese, French and Farsi.

Breast cancer

The UK incidence and mortality for breast cancer is the highest in the world (McPherson *et al*, 2000). The incidence of breast cancer increases with age, doubling about every ten years until the menopause when the rate of increase slows dramatically (McPherson *et al*, 2000). Of the 30,000 women diagnosed with breast cancer in England and Wales each year, 13,000 die . There is a 75% chance of surviving five years or more if the tumour is detected early (NHS Breast screening — The facts).

The peak time for developing breast cancer is between the ages of fifty and sixty-four (Umeh and Rogan-Gibson, 2001). In the UK, one woman in seventy will develop ovarian cancer compared to one woman in twelve developing breast cancer at some point in their lifetime (Briant, 1999). Hine (2001) points out that the incidence for lung cancer is becoming a very close second to breast cancer in women and, indeed, the lung cancer rates in women are rising while those in men are falling. Nearly 33% of cancer cases and 20% of cancer deaths in women are attributed to breast cancer, representing 30,000 cases and 11,000 deaths every year. However, around 65% of women survive breast cancer for at least five years after diagnosis. The survival rate for breast cancer is now more encouraging than it was thirty years ago as then only about 50% of women would survive, compared with around 70% today (Telegraph, 2001a). The annual spend by the NHS on breast cancer is £150 million.

The risk factors for developing breast cancer are a family history, a long menstrual and reproductive history, and poor socio-economic status (Deuster, 1996). A long menstrual and reproductive history equates to early age at menarche, late age at menopause, never having had children or a late age at first birth (Woods and Mitchell, 1997).

Early onset of periods also increase a woman's risk of developing breast cancer. Women who had started their periods at fifteen were at only two thirds the risk of premenopausal breast cancer compared with women whose periods had started at eleven. The risk decreased by 7% for every year that periods were delayed.

(Eaton, 2002, p. 386)

Women who have a natural menopause after the age of fifty-five are twice as likely to develop breast cancer than women who experience it prior to the age of forty-five. Women who have their first child after the age of thirty have twice the risk of a woman who has their first child before the age of twenty. The highest risk group, according to McPherson *et al* (2000) is women who have their first child over the age of thirty-five.

A recent study conducted in the Southern General Hospital in Glasgow, found that women from deprived areas were more likely to develop oestrogen receptor negative tumours which are seen as a more aggressive form of breast cancer as they are more difficult to treat and do not respond to Tamoxifen (BBC News Online, 2002a).

Where there is a family history of breast cancer, if a woman's mother or sister has had breast cancer, her risk of developing breast cancer is between two and three times greater than that of the general population. A woman who has had cancer in one breast has up to five times increased risk of developing cancer in the remaining breast, compared with the general population (Woods and Mitchell, 1997; McPherson *et al*, 2000).

McPherson *et al* (2000) state an additional risk factor is obesity. Obese postmenopausal women have twice the risk of developing breast cancer than obese pre-menopausal women. Naismith (1999, p. 2) offers the following explanation for this:

Hormones can predispose to a cancer by stimulating cell

proliferation, mainly in their normal target tissues. Obese women generally have higher levels of available oestrogen than normal weight women, which might explain the higher risk of postmenopausal breast cancer associated with obesity.

It has also been noted that there is a higher risk of developing breast cancer for women living in the South of England and Wales than in the North of the UK. The risk also appears higher in more affluent women (NHS, *Breast screening — The facts*).

The earlier breast cancer is diagnosed the better the prognosis. In the UK, the health message is to become breast aware so that any changes can be readily identified and medical opinion sought. Breast awareness involves women getting to know the appearance of their own breasts by looking and feeling them at a time that is best suited to them as an individual. This is important for all women from their mid-twenties onwards. The NHS Breast Screening Programme (1994) advised a five-point plan:

- know what is normal for you
- look and feel
- know what changes to look for (lump, thickening, pain, nipple discharge)
- report any changes without delay
- attend for breast screening if fifty or over.

Bearing in mind that 50% of breast cancer cases are in women over the age of sixty-five, it is imperative that women in their fifties and over become breast aware and attend for breast screening. Briant (1999) states that barriers to being breast aware can be attributed to embarrassment, reluctance to touch one's own breasts, lack of knowledge, fear, poor memory and lack of confidence in it as a screening technique. Rather worryingly, Briant (1999) reports research that demonstrates that nurses are poor at teaching breast awareness to older women.

Blamey *et al* (2000) state that there is no empirical evidence to suggest that clinical examination or teaching breast self-examination are effective tools in the early detection of breast cancer. However, they report that randomised controlled trials have demonstrated that screening by mammography can significantly reduce the mortality from breast cancer by up to 40% of those who attend.

Kmietowicz (2002a) cites figures from WHO which state that in the age group, fifty to sixty-eight, the death rate can be reduced by

35% through early detection using mammography. The NHS document, *Breast screening — The facts,* states that over 85% of breast cancers are diagnosed without undergoing the stress of an operation. The NHS has been offering screening for breasts and cervix since the late 1980s and the DoH (1999) states that regular screening for women aged fifty to sixty-four for breast cancer will eventually save up to an estimated 1,250 lives each year in the UK. The frequency of screening is dependent on the age of the woman. Blamey *et al* (2000) suggest that women between the ages of fifty and sixty years should attend for screening every two to three years and those under fifty more frequently.

Whether women participate regularly in breast awareness and screening is related to their own health beliefs. In the health belief model women who believe that they are susceptible to breast cancer or that breast cancer is a serious threat, or who believe that being breast aware or attending for breast screening is being proactive in terms of their health, will participate in these activities. Women who perceive little or no gain from them will not (Umeh and Rogan-Gibson, 2001). Dibble *et al* (1997, p. 47) relate this behaviour to the theory of reasoned action. They state that:

> *According to the theory of reasoned action, people make rational decisions about engaging in particular behaviours based upon available information. For example, intention to participate in breast screening is determined primarily by two factors: the woman's attitude to the breast cancer screening procedure and the social normative influence of the people who are important in her life.*

Blamey *et al* (2000) add three factors affecting whether women attend for breast screening: level of encouragement from their GP; their knowledge of screening programmes; views and experience of family and friends. An American randomised controlled trial conducted by Somkin *et al* (1997) found that women who received reminder letters were more likely to complete mammography and cervical smear screening than those that received the usual care.

Sheikh and Ogden (1998) report reasons why women do not attend for breast screening as being related to avoidance, fear and denial. Lauver *et al* (1995) provide some insight into why some women delay seeking help once they discover a problem with their breast. They state that between 20% and 26% of women delay at least two to three months after finding symptoms due to fear and anxiety. Yet the same fear and anxiety will make other women seek help promptly. Lauver *et al* (1995) add that conflicting role and time commitments are primary barriers in seeking help and that if health care services were at more convenient times women may not delay in seeking advice.

There is evidence that women are becoming more knowledgeable about breast cancer. Meric *et al* (2002) relate the findings of a recent survey which demonstrates that breast cancer is one of the most common health topics for users of the Internet. Between 40% and 54% of patients gain access to medical information in this way and this information is said to affect their choice of treatment. They also report Berland *et al*'s (2001) study that demonstrated that the information provided on web sites about breast cancer were more likely to be complete and accurate compared to other conditions.

Cervical cancer

Cervical cancer is a common cancer affecting women world-wide. In England and Wales the incidence figures for 1997 were approximately ten women in every 100,000 developing cervical cancer, with five women in every 100,000 dying as a result (Shepherd *et al*, 2000). Women in Northwest England have a 33% greater risk of developing cervical cancer than the national average (DoH, 1999). According to the NHS Cancer Screening Programme website, the UK has the second highest recorded incidence of cervical cancer in the European Union and it is the twelfth most common cause of cancer death in the UK.

Our Healthier Nation (DoH 1999) states that the human papilloma virus (HPV) is associated with about 3,000 cases of cervical cancer and more than 1,000 deaths each year. The NHS Cancer Screening Programme documents state that HPV is linked with 95% of cases of cervical cancer. According to Shepherd *et al* (2000), the most significant risk factor in developing cervical cancer is contracting HPV, a fact reinforced by Moreno *et al* (2002). The prevalence of HPV in cervical cancer is estimated at 99.7%. The HPV is sexually transmitted and can cause cervical cancer between five and thirty years after contracting the initial infection (Shepherd *et al*, 2000). Having multiple sexual partners who do not use condoms increases the risk of contracting HPV. Shepherd *et al* (2000) note that girls of fifteen who have sexual intercourse have twice the risk of contracting HPV and developing cervical cancer than those who had their first sexual encounter after the age of twenty.

Other risk factors associated with cervical cancer are smoking, the use of the contraceptive pill and chlamydia infection. Shepherd *et al* (2000) suggest that the trend in women in lower socio-economic groups developing cervical cancer could be explained by the higher cigarette smoking rates in this group. Smokers are regarded as being at double the risk of those who do not smoke (NHS Cancer Screening Programme).

A recent study conducted by the WHO's International Agency for Research has found that prolonged use of the oral contraceptive pill increases the risk of cervical cancer up to four times, but only in women who carry HPV. In the UK, HPV is present in about 30% of all women in their twenties (Dyer, 2002a). Importantly, Dyer (2002a) quotes a spokesperson from the Family Planning Association as saying:

> *The overall likelihood of getting cervical cancer in the UK is low, whether you use the pill or not... The benefits of using oral contraception outweigh the risks for the vast majority of women. The pill reduces the risk of cancer of the ovaries and the womb.*

Skegg (2002) asserts that HPV alone is not a sufficient cause of cervical cancer and that other factors are also associated, such as: infectious agents, for example, chlamydia; high parity; cigarette smoking; and oral contraception.

Cervical cancer is readily detectable and has a treatable precursor stage, which means that cervical screening is extremely valuable in preventing cervical cancer from developing. In the UK, cervical screening has been offered since the late 1980s. According to the DoH (1999), cervical screening prevents up to 3,900 cases of cervical cancer every year.

They state that the number of women dying from cervical cancer has fallen by 25% since 1994; the mortality rate reduced by 60% since 1988 and an estimated 1,300 lives saved in 1997 through cervical screening. Cervical screening is directly responsible for a 42% drop in the incidence of cervical cancer between 1988 and 1987 and it is estimated that regular attendance can prevent 80–90% of cervical cancers developing (The NHS Cancer Screening Programme).

The NHS Cancer Screening Programme adds that almost 50% of the 3,500 new cases of cervical cancer in the UK occur in women who have never had a smear test, and they conclude that the biggest risk factor is actually non-attendance for cervical screening. The following table (*Table 7.4*) demonstrates the effectiveness of cervical screening.

Table 7.4: Effectiveness of cervical screening

Interval of cervical screening	Age at screening	Reduction in cumulative incidence of cervical cancer
Single screen	40 years	20%
Five-yearly screening	20–64 years	83.6%
Three-yearly screening	20–64 years	91.2%
Annual screening	20–64 years	93.3%

From the above figures, it should be apparent that the regular attendance for cervical screening is imperative to prevent the development of cervical cancer. The NHS Cancer Screening Programme advocates regular screening every three to five years as the best way of detecting changes to the cervix early.

> *Research by Professor Sutton of the Institute of Public Health at Cambridge University found clear links between levels of deprivation and the uptake of screening. Middle-aged married women with cars were more likely to attend.*

(The NHS Cancer Screening Programme)

Khan *et al* (1999) conducted a qualitative study using focus groups and in-depth semi-structured interviews with fifteen American adolescents with the aim of investigating how adolescent girls understand and receive cervical smear screening and to identify any barriers to compliance. Khan *et al* found that the girls had little knowledge of cervical smears, however, they were aware that cervical smears were important in the prevention and early detection of cervical cancer. Perceived barriers were pain (n=13), embarrassment (n=10), fear of finding a problem or of the unknown (n=11), denial or perceived invincibility (n=6), and a lack of knowledge (n=4).

Patnick (2001) reports that some women report that they are apprehensive about attending because of a perception that it will be painful (n=12%) and 22% stated that embarrassment was a factor. It is important to be able to reassure women that while the procedure may be a little uncomfortable, it is of short duration and the test can be conducted by a female practitioner. It is also known that some women in ethnic minority groups are reluctant to attend for cervical screening. For example, 50% of Bangladeshi women are less likely to attend than other women in the UK (DoH, 1999).

It is important to advise women who are post-menopausal that they still require cervical smear tests to ensure that their cervix remains healthy. Furthermore, some women who have had hysterectomies believe that they no longer have to attend for screening. This is not always the case as not all women who have had hysterectomies have had their cervix removed and it is important that they check with their GP or practice nurse.

Sexually transmitted infections

In England in 1996, there were 300,000 cases of sexually transmitted infections (STIs), which included: cases of genital warts (n=50,000 plus); non-specific urethritis (n=50,000 plus); proven chlamydia (n=30,000 plus); genital herpes (n=15,000 plus); and gonorrhoea (n=10,000 plus) (Carne, 1998). Midgely (2002) reports that cases of gonorrhoea have increased since 1995 in men by 74%, and in women by 75%, and that syphilis in men (3/4 of heterosexual men) has risen by 211% in the past three years. Adolescents are most at risk of acquiring STIs (Shrier *et al*, 2001). Increasing attention is being paid to the incidence of STIs in adolescents, as the highest rates of gonorrhoea and chlamydia are in men between the ages of twenty and twenty-four and in women between the ages of sixteen and nineteen (Gilson and Mindel, 2001).

The risk factors associated with contracting a STI are having multiple sexual partners, unprotected sex and having partners who are at high risk of having a STI (Shrier *et al*, 2001). These factors are related to engaging in risky sexual behaviours, the development of which is associated with depression, and low self-esteem (Bennett and Bauman, 2000). Self-esteem is the perception of self-worth or positive feelings about oneself and is an important indicator of mental health (Shrier *et al*, 2001). Shrier *et al* (2001) conducted a longitudinal study of 3,192 American boys and 3,391 girls to assess the relationship of depressive symptoms and low self-esteem with condom non-use and self reported history of STI. They found that depressive symptoms were associated with condom non-use by boys and a history of STIs in both girls and boys. Boys with the highest level of depressive symptoms had more than three times the odds of ever developing a STI. Depressive symptoms were not associated with non-use of condoms in girls.

> *Condom use is a male-controlled method of sexually transmitted disease prevention and may have little to do with individual factors of female sexual partners.*
>
> (Shrier *et al*, 2001, p. 185)

Shrier *et al* (2001) conclude that young people with depression may have high risk partners because of feelings of worthlessness or impaired social functioning and, furthermore, that sexually active young people with depressive symptoms are more likely to engage in condom non-use and be diagnosed with STIs than their counterparts who are not depressed. They also noted that very frequent alcohol use had an effect on increasing unsafe sexual practices.

The Action for Adolescent Health (WHO, 1997) stipulates that behavioural patterns acquired in adolescence will last a lifetime. The adolescent years are an opportune time to prevent the onset of health-damaging behaviours and their future repercussions. Prevention and control of STIs involve three basic strategies. Firstly, reducing the risk of transmission by condom use; secondly, the rate of changes in sexual partners and; thirdly, reducing the period of infection (and thereby spread) in individuals by screening (Catchpole, 2001).

Human papilloma virus (HPV)

There are various types of HPV and they are categorised according to whether they are high or low risk on the basis of whether they cause cancer changes of the genital tract, principally cervical cancer. Types 6 and 11 are considered low risk but types 16 and 18 are high risk as these are the types most commonly associated with cervical cancer (Gilson and Mindel, 2001). Types 6 and 11 are associated with 90% of genital warts, of which, 72,233 cases of a first attack were diagnosed in 1999. This represents a 25% increase in men and 28% increase in women since 1993 (Gilson and Mindel, 2001). Untreated genital warts are associated with cervical cancer (DoH, 2001g).

The primary prevention of contracting HPV, chlamydia and the risk of developing cervical cancer is by the use of condoms during sexual intercourse. However, changing behaviour in this regard is complex. Shepherd *et al* (2000) state that providing information alone is not sufficient to change behaviour. They suggest that small group discussions, chaired by a knowledgeable peer, in which a variety of health promotion media are used, is more effective.

Chlamydia

The DoH (2001g) report that findings from a 1999 survey found that the majority of people questioned were unaware of what chlamydia was. Chlamydia is the most common and curable sexually transmitted infection in the UK (Oakeshott *et al*, 1998). The highest rates are found in sixteen to nineteen-year-old women (791 per 100,000) and in twenty to twenty-four-year-old men (465 per 100,000). In 1999, there were 56,855 patients with uncomplicated chlamydia infections seen in genito-urinary medicine clinics, representing a 61% increase since 1996 (DoH, 2001g). The actual prevalence of chlamydia is actually unknown but it is estimated to be as high as 10% of all people under the age of twenty (Thompson *et al*, 2001).

Midgely (2002) states that it is thought that one in ten individuals could be infected without being aware and that the greatest rise in incidence of the infection is in girls aged sixteen to nineteen years of age (141% rise). Kane *et al* (2001) report a geographical variation in incidence. In 1999, the incidence rates were highest for both men and women in London. Outside London, the highest rates for men were in the Northwest and Trent areas and lowest in Wales and Northern Ireland. The highest rates for women, outside London, were in Trent, Yorkshire and Northwest regions of England and lowest in Scotland and Northern Ireland.

Sixty to eighty per cent of individuals with chlamydia are often asymptomatic (Hicks *et al*, 1999) which makes control of the infection more difficult. Kane *et al* (2001) report that it is estimated that 50% of infected men and 70% of infected women have no symptoms and are unaware that they are passing the infection on to their partner. When symptoms are present they manifest by a purulent discharge, dysuria and urethritis (Josefson, 2001b).

There is evidence from Sweden and the USA that screening for chlamydia is effective and cost-effective (Oakeshott *et al*, 1998; Pimenta *et al*, 2002). Targeted screening in the USA achieved a reduction in 50% of cases of pelvic inflammatory disease (Bower, 1998). In the USA, sexually active girls are screened every six to twelve months (Hopkins, 1998).

There have been pilot schemes set up to examine the feasibility, acceptability and cost-effectiveness of screening for chlamydia in Portsmouth and the Wirral (Kane *et al*, 2001). These pilot sites use an opportunist screening mechanism which means that any time a female who meets the inclusion criteria attends a healthcare setting they are offered screening for chlamydia regardless of the reason for their initial attendance. The inclusion criteria are that they are either under twenty-five and sexually active or over twenty-five and have a new sexual partner or have had more than two sexual partners in the past year. The pilot sites are targeting women only as once a chlamydia infection is diagnosed, partner notification is carried out. Diagnosis of chlamydia has increased by 18% to 60,000 cases in 2000, which means that a case is diagnosed every ten minutes (Akid 2002). The primary screening test uses a sample of urine and treatment consists of a fourteen-day course of antibiotics (Bower, 1998).

The rationale for targeting women for screening, according to Duncan and Hart (1999), is based on health benefits, cost-effectiveness and accessibility. Duncan *et al* (2001) state that the aim of chlamydia screening is to reduce the incidence of pelvic inflammatory disease and its concomitant complications. They state that the guidelines recommend that all partners of infected women in the past six months should be contacted and treated. Treating infected women without treating their infected partner(s) results in a high rate of re-infection, making notification and treatment of partners essential (Gilson and Mindel, 2001).

Duncan *et al* (2001) conducted a qualitative study involving seventeen women with current or recent chlamydial infection. The findings demonstrated that these women had three primary concerns. Firstly, concerns after hearing the diagnosis related to feelings of stigma; secondly, worry about their future reproductive health; and thirdly, anxiety associated with notifying their partners. Duncan *et al* (2001, p. 198) offer the following implications arising from their study:

> *Firstly, information given to women before screening should seek to normalise and destigmatise chlamydial infection to reduce the negative psychological impact of a positive diagnosis. Secondly, although it was clear that the information given to women by staff served to lessen, if not eradicate, stigma, disclosure of the condition to others remained a source of anxiety (specifically, that others would react badly). This anxiety may be exacerbated if women feel unable to access their usual support network.*

Thus, support services should be available if required. Women attending a genitourinary medicine clinic highlighted the important role of health visitors in providing advice and reassurance. Given the uncertainties associated with chlamydial infection and that reassurance about one factor can increase anxiety about another, staff outside specialised services may require guidance in providing support to women diagnosed with infection. Finally, the chief medical officer's report recommends that women with positive diagnoses should be referred to genitourinary medicine clinics for support and advice about telling partners. It acknowledges that some patients may not take up referral and that education is required to destigmatise genitourinary medicine services.

Since individuals can have chlamydia and not be aware of it the infection is often untreated. The effects of untreated chlamydia are serious for both men and women. In women, untreated chlamydia can lead to pelvic inflammatory disease, ectopic pregnancy and infertility. Half the cases of pelvic inflammatory disease in England and Wales are attributed to chlamydia and pelvic inflammatory disease is the leading cause of infertility and chronic pelvic pain. Even one episode of pelvic inflammatory disease can have a 20% chance of leaving the woman infertile and the risk increases double-fold with each subsequent episode. Some 40% of ectopic pregnancies are attributed to chlamydia. Chlamydia can also cause miscarriage and infection in new-born babies (Kane *et al*, 2001), resulting in neonatal ophthalmia and genital tract colonisation (Thompson *et al*, 2001). In men, untreated chlamydia infection causes epididymo-orchitis (Thompson *et al*, 2001).

Chlamydia can be prevented and controlled by the use of a condom during sexual intercourse. Kane *et al* (2001) report the results of a poll carried out by the Health Education Authority in 1997. These indicated that only 26% of sixteen to twenty-four-year-olds had heard about chlamydia and, of these 26%, only 32% of them knew what the symptoms and effects were. Kane *et al* (2001) remark that the prevention and control of chlamydia infection would have a major impact on the reproductive health of women. It would also have a considerable financial effect, as conservative estimates are that the cost of diagnosis and treatment of chlamydia and its complications cost £50 million every year in the UK.

In the Scottish Health Education Population Survey (HEBS,

2000), 63% of respondents agreed with the statement that they would not have sex with a new partner without a condom, however, 30% felt that buying condoms was an embarrassing experience. Men were more likely to have changed their sexual behaviour as a result of perceived risk of HIV/AIDS; 18% of men compared to 12% of women. It was noted that younger age groups were the most likely group to have changed their sexual behaviour. This was particularly noticeable in the sixteen to thirty-four-year-old age group; 28% compared to 15% overall. In line with the Health Belief Model, those who see themselves at greater risk also appear to be more likely to adopt preventative strategies (HEBS, 2000).

Coleman and Ingham (1999) also advocate that providing information and increasing awareness of contraception requires discussions with young people so that they can identify with the benefits in its use. Coleman and Ingham (1999) conducted semi-structured interviews with fifty-six young men and women with the aim of exploring the number of explanations as to why people experience difficulties in talking about contraception with their partners. They found that the most prominent explanation was concern that their partner would react negatively and make assumptions that by talking about contraception there was an intention for intercourse and initiating condom use may imply that they had a sexually transmissible infection. When they explored this further, they found that rather than seeing it negatively, partners stated that they would view it positively as an act of showing care and respect.

Coleman and Ingham (1999) concluded that young people should be encouraged to carry condoms at all times as, by their own volition in interviews, intercourse occurred predominantly unexpectedly.

MacPhail and Campbell (2001, p. 1615) add to the debate about young people carrying condoms. They state that:

> *A high regard for preservation of reputation means that young women adhere to social definitions of sexual encounters as initiated by men, against female resistance. Women, therefore, often do not have condoms available and make few efforts to gain knowledge of their partner's sexual histories, as this would be tantamount to admitting to themselves and society that they plan to engage in sex. In addition, women often avoid carrying condoms due to the negative reputations and labels associated with women who actively seek sex.*

Mawer (1999) states that visible marketing can significantly increase condom use (but not sexual activity) for high-risk women.

Teenage pregnancy

According to the Social Exclusion Unit (1999), Britain has the highest teenage pregnancy rate in western Europe. The average age for commencement of sexual intercourse is said to be seventeen years of age, which compares with figures from 1960 of twenty-one for females and twenty for men. It is estimated that between 30% and 50% of teenagers do not use any form of contraception in their first sexual encounter, and over 25% of fourteen to fifteen-year-olds mistakenly believe that the contraceptive pill protects against sexually transmitted infections (DoH, 2001g). There were 90,000 teenage conceptions in England and 56,000 resulted in live births. The actual conception figures vary across the UK but there is a direct correlation between high rates of teenage pregnancy and areas of high deprivation. Although the actual rate of teenage pregnancies has not altered over the last twenty years, it has markedly reduced in countries such as the Netherlands and France (Kiddy, 2002).

Birth rates among fifteen to nineteen-year-olds in the UK are seven times higher than those in the Netherlands where contraceptive use is more common (McKee, 1999). Ferriman (1999) reports that the UK teenage pregnancy rate is four times that of France. The teenage pregnancy rates in America are twice that of the UK (Foster, 2001). The rates of teenage pregnancies in thirteen to fifteen-year-olds in Scotland are higher than most other western European countries (HEBS, 2000).

Teenage pregnancy is usually associated with health inequalities and, according to Kiddy (2002), this perpetuates the myth that women get pregnant to gain access to housing and benefits. The reasons for teenage pregnancy are poorly understood. McLeod (2001) states that there are multiple reasons for the link between socio-economic deprivation and teenage pregnancies. In the 1990s, such deprivation explained more than 50% of local variation in rates of teenage pregnancy, more than double the amount in the 1980s (McLeod, 2001). McLeod suggests that as well as cultural and attitudinal differences to the concept of early motherhood, other factors include sexual risk taking, and employment and educational aspirations (p. 199).

Research studies demonstrate that adolescence is a time of experimentation and is strongly associated with taking risks (Kiddy, 2002). Dignan (2000) suggests the following reasons: non-use of contraception; overcrowded accommodation; unstable home life; lack of satisfaction at school; their own mothers were teenagers when they first conceived; low self-esteem and low self-worth. Foster (2001) points out that many adolescents have a heightened need to be loved. The commonest reason given by both sexes for early first intercourse was curiosity about what it would be like, followed by alcohol reducing inhibitions and peer pressure (Dickson *et al*, 1998).

There is a marked social class gradient, not only in respect of high rates in the more deprived social groups, but also in respect to high rates of pregnancies that go to term (Scottish Executive, 2001).

There is evidence to suggest that a society that is open about facts, beliefs and attitudes towards sex and sexuality and supports young people in making informed choices about their general and sexual health is a society which engenders positive personal and sexual relationships and delays the age of first intercourse.

(Scottish Executive, 2001, p. 46)

Indeed, in Holland, where the rates of teenage pregnancy are much lower, sex relationship education occurs in primary schools from a very early age (Illman, 2002).

Illman (2002) describes an initiative which was initially pioneered at Exeter University and now more than 100 schools take part. The initiative is called APAUSE, which stands for added power and understanding in sex education. The aim of APAUSE is to ensure that young people know how to avoid becoming pregnant in an unplanned way and to equip them with the skills necessary to deal with negative relationship situations. It involves school nurses and teachers working together in a classroom alongside an APAUSE trained pupil (peer educators) and together they run sessions for pupils about sexuality, relationships and contraception. The initiative is targeted at young teenagers, as it is known that teenagers who have sex for the first time before the age of sixteen are unlikely to use contraception. Illman (2002) reports that 25% of young females and 30% of young males have sex under the age of sixteen although the average age of first intercourse for both sexes is sixteen years of age.

Of those who did have their first sexual intercourse between the ages of thirteen and fourteen, two in five males and four in five females admit that they wished that they had waited longer. Illman suggests that involving peer educators is more likely to have a positive effect and to dismiss some misconceptions such as, 'all sixteen-year-olds do it'. Peer educators are respected, states Illman, because they are seen to be older than the pupils they are teaching, but not too old to be dismissed as having no idea as to what it is really like.

In 1999, there were approximately 174,000 termination of pregnancies performed in England and Wales. The highest rates were seen in women in their twenties (DoH, 2001g). Teenagers who choose not to terminate their pregnancies face a range of responses from their family and friends. If these are negative, the young person can experience both mental and physical health problems and become socially isolated (DoH, 2001g; Whitehead, 2001). It can also have long-term adverse effects on education, employment and economic status (Kiddy, 2002). Payne (2001b) reports from an Irish Parliamentary Committee, which identified that 60% of babies born to teenage mothers are more likely to die than those born to older women.

The rationale provided for this are that teenage mothers are often single mothers who are more likely to live in poverty, less likely to finish their education and more likely to have poor social support.

Education is the most obvious tool to be used for reducing the number of teenage pregnancies. There are those who express concerns about sex education in schools as they believe that such education encourages earlier sexual activity. However, as Green (1998) reports, there is a growing body of evidence to suggest that the opposite is in fact the case and that it has been shown to delay the onset of sexual activity. The Government has set a target of reducing the number of teenage pregnancies in under eighteen-year-olds by half by 2010. Each area in England has a local teenage pregnancy strategy that is linked to a local funding mechanism. The strategies are based on four key areas: media campaigns, sex and relationship education, sexual health services and support for teenage parents (Kiddy, 2002).

There is a criticism that sex and relationship education occurs too late in schools. Most often it is placed within the curriculum in year ten when pupils are aged fourteen or fifteen, and there is evidence that sexual intercourse has been experienced prior to this age. Kiddy (2002) argues that there is a misconception that sex and relationship education promotes sexual behaviour, giving this as a rationale for the reticence in teaching younger children.

Kiddy (2002) reports that young women generally have low knowledge levels about emergency contraception and they acknowledge that they perceive barriers to using family planning clinics. Kiddy continues to report that almost 30% of those interviewed in a research study had not used any form of contraception.

The ten-year £60 million campaign for teenage pregnancies was launched in 1999. Teenage boys are targeted with the message that for any children they are responsible for fathering, they will be expected to contribute financially to their support. The campaign also emphasises how easy it is to get pregnant but how difficult it can be to be a parent, in particular a lone parent. The main thrust of the campaign is education and the expansion of effective and accessible NHS contraception services, particularly in areas where there are high rates of teenage pregnancy.

Ferriman (1999) reports that in England in 1997 there were 90,000 pregnant teenage girls; 8,000 of these were under sixteen and 2,200 were under fourteen years of age. She also cites Tessa Jowell, minister of public health, stating the following at the launch of the campaign:

> *The emphasis will be placed firmly on making sure that children know the facts about sex at an appropriate time and in an appropriate way and that they have the self-confidence to face down the pressure from partners or peers to have sex before they are ready.*

The targets set for reducing teenage pregnancies in England and Wales is 50% in teenagers under eighteen years of age by 2010. In Scotland, the target is a reduction of 20% in the pregnancy rate in thirteen to fifteen-year-olds by 2010 (McLeod, 2001).

Education should also include knowledge of emergency contraception. Mawer (1999) reports findings from a large randomised controlled trial, which found that administration of emergency contraception is safe, does not lead to overuse, and reduces pregnancies. Improving access to health education and contraceptive services is seen as fundamental in reducing teenage pregnancy (Churchill *et al*, 2000).

Suggested web resources

http://www.breasthealthnetwork.com/home/ Breast Health Network

http://www.cancerbacup.org.uk provides practical advice and support to cancer patients, their families and friends

http://commtechlab.msu.edu Breast cancer Lighthouse

http://www.nabco.org National Alliance of Breast Cancer Organisations
http://www.nature.com/nrc/ Nature Reviews Cancer
http://www.nejm.org/ *New England Journal of Medicine's* collection of breast cancer articles
http://www.sexhealth.org
http://www.wcn.org Women's cancer network

References

Akid M (2002) Let's talk about sex. *Nurs Times* **98**(12): 12–13

Bandolier (2002a) *Alcohol consumption and cancer risk.* http://www.jr2.ox.ac.uk/bandolier/booth/hliving/alccan.html (accessed March 2002)

Batty D, Thune I (2000) Does physical activity prevent cancer? *Br Med J* **321**: 1378–9

BBC News Online (2002a) *Breast cancer 'strikes most deprived'.* http://www.news.bbc.co.uk/l/hi/health/1883945.stm (accessed March 2002)

Bennett DL, Bauman A (2000) Adolescent mental health and risky sexual behaviour. *Br Med J* **321**: 251–2

Berland GK, Elliott MN, Morales LS, Algazy JI, Broder MS (2001) Health information on the internet: accessibility, quality and readability in English and Spanish. *JAMA* **285**(26) 12–21

Blamey RW, Wilson ARM, Patnick J (2000) Screening for breast cancer. *Br Med J* **321**: 689–93

Bower H (1998) Britain launches pilot screening for chlamydia. *Br Med J* **316**: 1477

Briant A (1999) *Breast awareness.* JCN Online 13(7) http://www.jcn.co.uk/ (accessed October 2002)

Cancer Working Group (1999) *Strategic Priorities in Cancer Research and Development.* http://www.doh.gov.uk/research/documents/rd3/cancer_fnal_report.pdf (accessed March 2002)

Carne C (1998) Sexually transmitted infections. *Br Med J* **317**: 129–32

Catchpole M (2001) Sexually transmitted infections: control strategies. *Br Med J* **322**: 1135–6

Churchill D, Allen J, Pringle M Hippisley-Cox J, Ebdon D, Macpherson M, Bradley S (2000) Consultation patterns and provision of contraception in general practice before teenage pregnancy: case-control study. *Br Med J* **321**: 486–9

Coleman LM, Ingham R (1999) Exploring young people's difficulties in talking about contraception: how can we encourage more discussion between partners? *Health Educ Res* **14**(6): 741–50

Department of Health, Social Services and Public Safety (2002) *Investing for Health.* http://www.dhsspsni.gov.uk/publications/ (accessed March 2002)

Deuster PA (1996) Exercise in the prevention and treatment of chronic disorders. *Women's Health Issues* **6**(6): 320–31

Dibble SL, Vanoni JM, Miaskowski C (1997) Women's attitudes toward breast cancer screening procedures: differences by ethnicity. *Women's Health Issues* **7**(1): 47–54

Dickson N, Paul C, Herbison P, Silva P (1998) First sexual intercourse: age; coercion, and later regrets by a birth cohort. *Br Med J* **316**: 29–33

Dignan K (2000) Teenage pregnancy. In: Kerr J, ed. *Community Health Promotion: Challenges for Practice.* Baillière Tindall, London: chapter 5

Department of Health (1999) *Saving Lives: Our Healthier Nation.* DoH, London

Department of Health (2001g) *The National Strategy for Sexual Health and HIV*. http://www.doh.gov.uk/nshs (accessed March 2002)

Duncan B, Hart G (1999) Sexuality and health: the hidden costs of screening for chlamydia trachomatis. *Br Med J* **318**: 931–3

Duncan B, Hart G, Scoular A, Bigrigg A (2001) Qualitative analysis of psychosocial impact of diagnosis of chlamydia trachomatis: implications for screening. *Br Med J* **322**: 195–9

Dyer O (2002a) WHO links long term pill use to cervical cancer. *Br Med J* **324**: 808

Eaton L (2002) Early periods and late childbearing increases risk of breast cancer, study confirms. *Br Med J* **324**: 386

Ferriman A (1999) England launches campaign on teenage pregnancies. *Br Med J* **318**: 1646

Foster HW (2001) Teen pregnancy reduction: A continuing challenge. *Women's Health in Primary Care* **4**(8): 521–6

Gilson RJC, Mindel A (2001) Sexually transmitted infections. *Br Med J* **322**: 1160–4

Green J (1998) The role of theory in evidence-based health promotion practice. *Health Educ Res* **15**(2): 125–9

Health Education Board for Scotland (2000) *Indicators for Health Education In Scotland: Summary of findings from the 1998 Health Education Population Survey*. HEBS, Edinburgh

Health Education Board for Scotland (2001) The Guide to Preventing Cancer. HEBS, Edinburgh http://www.hebs.scot.nhs.uk/topics/topicsection.cfm?topic-cancer&TxTCode=51&TxS

Hicks NR, Dawes M, Fleminger M, Goldman D, Hamling J, Hicks LJ (1999) Chlamydia infection in general practice. *Br Med J* **318**: 790–2

Hine D (2001) National perspective: United Kingdom. *Women's Health* **11**(4): 293–9

Hopkins J (1998) Regular chlamydia screening recommended. *Br Med J* **317**: 432

Illman J (2002) Good advice given with class. *Nurs Times* **98**(11): 27–8

Josefson D (2001b) Chlamydia increases risk of cervical cancer. *Br Med J* **322**: 71

Kane R, Khadduri R, Wellings K (2001) Screening for chlamydia among adolescents in the UK: a review of policy and practice. *Health Educ* **101**(3): 108–15

Khan JA, Chiou V, Allen JD (1999) Beliefs about Papanicolaou smears and compliance with Papanicolaou smear follow-up in adolescents. *Arch Pediatr Adolesc Med* **153**: 1046–54

Kiddy M (2002) Teenage pregnancy: whose problem? *Nurs Times* **98**(4): 36–37

Kinghorn G (2001) A sexual health and HIV strategy for England. *Br Med J* **323**: 243–4

Kmietowicz Z (2002a) WHO insists screening can cut breast cancer rates. *Br Med J* **324**: 695

Kono S (2001) All epidemiological evidence is important in colorectal cancer. *Br Med J* **322**: 611

Lauver D, Coyle M, Panchmatia B (1995) Women's reasons for and barriers to seeking care for breast cancer symptoms. *Women's Health Issues* **5**(1): 27–35

MacPhail C, Campbell C (2001) 'I think condoms are good but, I hate those things': condom use among adolescents and young people in a Southern African township. *Soc Sci Med* **52**: 1613–27

Mawer C (1999) Preventing teenage pregnancies, supporting teenage mothers. *Br Med J* **318**: 1713–4

McKee M (1999) Sex and drugs and rock and roll. *Br Med J* **318**: 1300–1

McLeod A (2001) Changing patterns of teenage pregnancy: population based study of small areas. *Br Med J* **323**: 199–202

McPherson K, Steel CM, Dixon JM (2000) Breast cancer — epidemiology, risk factors, and genetics. *Br Med J* **321**: 624–8

Meric F, Bernstam EV, Mirza NQ, Hunt KK, Ames FC, Ross MI, Kuerer, HM, Pollock RE, Musen MA, Singletary SE (2002) Breast cancer on the world wide web: cross sectional survey of quality of information and popularity of websites. *Br Med J* **324**: 577–81

Midgely C (2002) The price of casual sex. *The Times*, 29 January

Moreno V, Xavier Bosch F, Muroiz N, Meyer C, Shah KV, Walboomers J (2002) Effect of oral contraceptives on risk of cervical cancer in women with human papillomavirus infection: the IARC multicentric case-control study. *The Lancet* **359**: 1085–1086

Naismith D (1999) Diet and cancer — is there a link? JCN Online 13(9): 1–4. http://www.jcn.co.uk/backiss

Ness AR, Frankel SJ, Gunnell DJ, Smith GD (1999) Are we really dying for a tan? *Br Med J* **319**: 114–6

National Health Service (1994) *Breast Screening Programme 'Be Breast Aware'*. HMSO, London

NHS Breast Screening: The Facts. http://www.hpe.org.uk (accessed March 2002)

NHS Cancer Screening Programmes http://www.cancerscreening.nhs.uk (accessed April 2002)

Nicoll A, Catchpole M, Cliffe S, Hughes G, Simms I, Thomas D (1999) Sexual health of teenagers in England and Wales: analysis of national data. *Br Med J* **318**: 1321–2

Oakeshott P, Kerry S, Hay S, Hay P (1998) Opportunistic screening for chlamydial infection at time of cervical smear testing in general practice: prevalence study. *Br Med J* **316**: 351–2

Patnick J (2001) *Cervical Screening Programme Annual Review: Informed choice in cervical screening* http://www.cancerscreening.nhs.uk (accessed April 2002)

Payne D (2001b) Babies of teenage mothers 60% more likely to die. *Br Med J* **322**: 386

Pimenta J, Catchpole M, Gray M, Hopwood J, Randall S (2000) Screening for genital chlamydial infection. *Br Med J* **321**: 629–31

Scottish Executive (2001) *Health in Scotland*. http://www.show.scot.nhs.uk/publications (accessed February 2002)

Sheikh I, Ogden J (1998) The role of knowledge and beliefs in help seeking behaviour for cancer: a quantitative and qualitative approach. *Patient Education and Counseling* **35**: 35–42

Shepherd J, Peersman G, Weston R, Napuli I (2000) Cervical cancer and sexual lifestyle: a systematic review of health education interventions targeted at women. *Health Educ Res* **15**(6): 681–94

Shrier LA, Harris SK, Sternberg M, Beardslee WR (2001) Associations of depression, self-esteem and substance use with sexual risk among adolescents. *Prev Med* **33**: 179–89

Sikora K (1999) Cancer survival in Britain. *Br Med J* **319**: 461–2

Skegg DCG (2002) Oral contraceptives, parity and cervical cancer. *Lancet* **359**(9312): 1080–1

Social Exclusion Unit (1999) *Teenage pregnancy*. The Stationery Office, London

Somkin CP, Hiatt RA, Hurley LB (1997) The effect of patient and provider reminders on mammography and Papanicolaou smear screening in a large health maintenance organisation. *Arch Int Med* **157**: 1658–64

Telegraph (2001a) Suicide rate drops following painkiller sales law. http://www.dailytelegraph.co.uk (accessed May 2001).

Thompson C, Macdonald M, Sutherland S (2001) A family cluster of chalmydia trachomatis infection. *Br Med J* **322**: 1473–4

Umeh K, Rogan-Gibson J (2001) Perceptions of threat, benefits and barriers in breast self-examination amongst young asymptomatic females. *Br J Health Psychol* **6**: 361–72

Whitehead E (2001) Teenage pregnancy: on the road to social death. *Int J Nurs Stud* **38**: 437–46

WHO (1997) *Action for Adolescent Health: Towards a Common Agenda*. World Health Organization, Geneva

Woods MF, Mitchell ES (1997) Preventative Health Issues: The perimenopausal to mature years (45–64). In: Allen KM, Phillips JM, eds. *Women's Health: across the lifespan*. Lippincott, Philadelphia: chapter 5

Conclusion

Throughout the previous chapters reference has been made to how policies can influence the health of the population. There is a myriad of policies, which together serve this aim. These include: national screening programmes; road safety initiatives, including drink-driving campaigns and traffic-calming measures; immunisation programmes for influenza, rubella, mumps and tetanus; healthy eating advice; anti-smoking campaigns, including taxing cigarettes and banning tobacco advertising; food safety regulations, including the new Food Standards Agency; increasing child benefit or other social security benefits for those on low incomes; health and safety at work regulations; and improving the quality of housing (King's Fund, undated).

Obtaining health information and advice is reasonably easy, however, making everyone aware of where information can be accessed is another matter. In the previous chapters, a number of web addresses have been provided so that you, as a reader of this book, can disseminate this resource to those you encounter. As we have also seen, it is one thing to know and understand what to do in order to improve one's health, it is another to become motivated enough to make the difference and embrace the messages and change one's lifestyle and health behaviours. Below and *Table conclusion.1* are examples of tips and advice regarding healthy living.

Ten tips for better health

❖ Don't smoke. If you can, stop. If you can't, cut down.

❖ Follow a balanced diet with plenty of fruit and vegetables.

❖ Keep physically active.

❖ Manage stress by, for example, talking things through and making time to relax.

❖ If you drink alcohol, do so in moderation.

❖ Cover up in the sun, and protect children from sunburn.

❖ Practise safer sex.

❖ Take up cancer screening opportunities.

❖ Be safe on the roads: follow the Highway Code.

(Source: Liam Donaldson Chief Medical Officer: DoH,1999)

Bandolier's (2002c) tips to incorporate exercise into your lifestyle:

- take the stairs instead of lifts or elevators
- if you work in a large office, walk to talk to your colleagues, rather than picking up the phone
- if you use buses, get off a stop or two earlier and walk
- don't worry about finding a car park next to the supermarket or shop entrance. By the time you have found a close car park you could have walked from a further, empty and less stressful place!
- for normal amounts of shopping or other errands use a bicycle instead of the car, saving you money and the hassle of finding a parking space. If you live in a town you will probably save time and if you live in the country you can enjoy the countryside
- if you have a cordless phone, walk and talk.

Table Conclusion.1: Summary of advice on healthy living (Bandolier, 2002b)

	Advice	Rationale
1.	Eat wholegrain foods (bread, rice or pasta) on four occasions a week.	This will reduce the chance of having almost any cancer by 40%. Given that cancer affects about one in three of us in a lifetime, that's good advice.
2.	Don't smoke. If you do smoke, stop. Nicotine patches, gum or inhaler won't help much, and acupuncture won't help at all. Cut down to below five cigarettes a day and leave long portions of the day without a cigarette.	Try to reduce your smoking, as there is a profound dose-response (the more you smoke, the more likely you are to have cancer, or heart or respiratory disease).
3.	Eat at least five portions of vegetables and fruit a day, and especially tomatoes (including ketchup), red grapes and the like as well as salad all year.	This protects against a whole variety of different nasty things: it reduces the risk of stroke dramatically; it reduces the risk of diabetes considerably and it will reduce the risk of coronary heart disease and cancer.
4.	Use Benecol instead of butter or margarine.	It really does reduce cholesterol, and reducing cholesterol will reduce the risk of heart attack and stroke even in those whose cholesterol is not particularly high.
5.	Drink alcohol regularly, but in moderation. Having a day without alcohol won't hurt either.	Suggested helpful in reducing the risk of cardiovascular disease.
6.	Eat fish.	Eating fish once a week won't stop you having a heart attack in itself, but it reduces the likelihood of your dying from it by half.
7.	Take a multivitamin tablet every day, but be sure that it is one with at least 200 micrograms of folate.	The evidence is that this can substantially reduce chances of heart disease in some individuals, and it has been shown to reduce colon cancer by over 85%. It may reduce the likelihood of developing dementia. Folate is essential in any woman contemplating pregnancy because it will reduce the chance of some birth defects.
8.	Drink no more than four cups of coffee a day. If you are pregnant or have high blood pressure, coffee is best minimised.	Drinking four cups of coffee a day is likely to reduce your chances of getting colon cancer and Parkinson's disease.
9.	Get more breathless more often. You don't have to go to a gym or be an Olympic marathon runner. Simply walking a mile a day, or taking reasonable exercise three times a week (enough to make you sweat or glow) will substantially reduce the risk of heart disease. If you walk, don't dawdle. Make a brisk pace.	One of the benefits of regular exercise is that it strengthens bones and keeps them strong. Breaking a hip when elderly is a very serious thing.
10.	Check your height and weight on a chart to see if you are overweight for your height. Your body mass index is the weight in kilograms divided by the height in metres squared: for preference it should be below 24. If you are overweight, lose it.	Losing weight has many benefits and there is no good evidence on simple ways to lose weight that work. Crash diets don't work. Take it one step at a time, do the things that are possible now and combine some calorie limitation with increased exercise.

Table Conclusion.2: Top ten reasons to take a health supplement from the Health Supplements Information Service

1. Pre-conceptual and pregnant women: Scientific evidence shows that folic acid supplement prior to conception and during the first twelve weeks of pregnancy can significantly reduce the incidence of neural tube defects in the foetus, such as spina bifida.

2. Vegetarians and vegans: Those on vegetarian or vegan diets can benefit from vitamin B12, vitamin D, calcium, iron and zinc supplementation.

3. Smokers: Each cigarette smoked depletes some vitamin C. Vitamin C is an antioxidant which neutralises potentially damaging free radicals in the body. Studies indicate that smokers require double the amount of vitamin C compared to non-smokers. In France and Canada higher RDAs have been established for smokers.

4. Athletes: When undertaking a rigorous exercise routine, it may be useful to increase the intake of antioxidants (beta-carotene, bioflavonoids, vitamin C and vitamin E) as there is an increased production of free radicals in the body. Antioxidants neutralise potentially damaging free radicals. Athletes also need to consume adequate amounts of minerals, such as calcium for healthy bones.

5. Elderly: The over sixty-fives are less efficient at absorbing essential vitamins and minerals, which can result in the immune response being compromised. Supplements of vitamin B12, C and E can therefore be helpful. The Government currently recommends that people over sixty-five take a vitamin D supplement.

6. Lactating women: Those who consume low levels of calcium can benefit from a calcium supplement of 1000mg a day, as their requirement for calcium increases during lactation. Lactating women who habitually cover up their skin for cultural or religious reasons or don't eat fortified fat spreads or animal products, a daily 10mg vitamin D supplement should be taken to assist in their child's formation of healthy bones and teeth. However, before taking any supplements, lactating women should always check with their GP first.

7. Young children: Children can go through 'fussy eating' periods when they may not receive all the nutrients they need. A multivitamin specially aimed at children can be beneficial at these times.

8. Convalescents: Convalescents are less likely to eat a balanced diet and since they may also need extra help to aid recovery, health supplementation can be beneficial. The average number of days of illness in long-term patients was shown to be reduced by 50% in a year when given a multivitamin supplement.

9. People with busy and stressful lives: People with busy lifestyles and those who are trying to lose weight may sometimes skip meals and find it difficult to always eat a balanced diet, including the recommended five daily portions of fruit and vegetables. A daily multivitamin can help ensure essential nutrients are provided at these times.

10. People on restrictive dietary regimes: People whose diets are restricted, such as those who have food allergies, eg. wheat allergy, may benefit from taking a daily multivitamin supplement.

(Source: http://www.hsis.org/press/000724.htm)

The future is not the result of choices among alternative paths offered;
It's a place that is created,
Created first in the mind and will
Created next in activity
The future is not some place we are going to
But one we are creating
The paths to it are not found but made
The activity of making them changes the maker and the destiny.

(Anon)

Suggested web resources

http://www.cancerbacup.org.uk

http://www.doh.gov.uk/research/index.htm

http://www.fons.org/ Foundation of Nursing Studies is an independent charity which is dedicated to supporting nurses to put nursing research into practice to improve patient care

http://www.kingsfund.org.uk The King's Fund is an independent charitable foundation whose goal is to improve health, especially in London. They focus on tackling health inequalities and social injustice; enabling health and social care staff and organisations to work in partnership, across traditional boundaries; promote cultural diversity in health; and encourage patient and wider public involvement in health and health care

http://www.medisearch.co.uk (accessed October 2002)

http://www.nelh-pc.nhs.uk National Primary Care Research and Development Centre. A multi- disciplinary centre established in 1995, which is dedicated to excellence in primary care research. The purpose of NPCRDC is to improve primary and community health care in the NHS through the generation, dissemination and application of knowledge and ideas relevant to the funding, organisation and delivery of health services. NPCRDC, which is funded by the Department of Health, has its main base at the University of Manchester.

http://www.npcrdc.man.ac.uk

http://ww.nhsdirect.nhs.uk NHS Direct Online provides information about healthy living and health care as well as a database of information for patients and the public on a variety of conditions. The database contains contact details for major national organisations and self-help groups and details of evaluated patient information leaflets and booklets on treatment choices. It also contains a guide to the NHS

http://www.nmap.ac.uk an Internet resource for nurses, midwives and allied health professionals

http://www.nursepractitioner.org.uk This site aims to inform and network practice nurses, links and discussion sites

http://www.show.scot.nhs.uk/

http://www.wales.nhs.uk

http://www.nelh.nhs.uk National electronic Library for Health

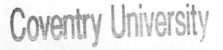

http://www.jr2.ox.ac.uk/bandolier/booth/booths/women.html Provides information on women's health issues, such as; breast cancer, sexual health, pregnancy and childbirth, menopause and osteoporosis, coronary heat disease, ovarian cancer

References

Bandolier (2002b) Bandolier's summary of advice on healthy living.
http://www.jr2.oc.ac.uk/bandolier/booth/hliving/10steps.html (accessed March 2002)
Bandolier (2002c) *Starting to exercise.*
http://www.jr2.ox.ac.uk/bandolier/booth/hliving/startoex.html (accessed March 2002)
Department of Health (1999) *Saving Lives: Our Healthier Nation.* DoH, London
King's Fund (undated) *Public Health and Public Values.* Kings Fund, London

Index